Wendy Talks Menopause

WENDY NAUMOVSKI

Wendy Talks Menopause

**What No One Told Me
What I Learned &
How You Can Thrive**

First published in 2026 by Dean Publishing
PO Box 119
Mt. Macedon, Victoria, 3441
Australia
deanpublishing.com

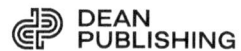

Copyright © Wendy Naumovski

All rights reserved. No part of this publication may be reproduced, stored in a retrieval system or transmitted in any way or by any means, electronic, mechanical, photocopying, recording or otherwise, without the prior written permission of the author and publisher.

Cataloguing-in-Publication Data
National Library of Australia

Title: Wendy Talks Menopause
ISBN: 978-0-648995-74-6
Category: Self-Help/Menopause

Photographer, front cover – Daniel Mostyn.

The views and opinions expressed in this book are those of the author and do not necessarily reflect the official policy or position of any other agency, publisher, organisation, employer, medical body, psychological body, or company. Assumptions made in the analysis are not reflective of the position of any entity other than the author(s) — and, these views are always subject to change, revision, and rethinking at any time.

The author, publisher or organisations are not to be held responsible for misuse, reuse, recycled and cited and/or uncited copies of content within this book by others.

The ideas within this book are based on the author's experience and are not intended to replace any professional advice or diagnose or treat any health or mental issues. This book is not intended to treat health or psychological issues but act as a reflective and inspiring resource for personal development.

This book isn't just for women in the thick of menopause. It's for the next generation too.

To my daughters, Nataya, Caprice and Armani, this is for you.

I want you to read these words not because you're in this season, but because one day you will live it. And when that time comes, I want you to be ready. Not blindsided. Not confused. Not angry at your body or your mind for changing into someone you barely recognise.

You live in a world that's already spinning faster than your nervous system can keep up with. Constant notifications. Pressure to keep up. Expectations to be perfect, productive, polite. If you can start early – learn how to slow down, breathe deeply, take care of your gut, your cycle, your stress – you can enter this phase of life with tools, prepared.

I want you to see menopause not as the end of youth, but the beginning of something sacred.

A new chapter of wisdom. A deeper sense of knowing yourself. A time where you stop saying yes to everyone else, and finally say yes to you.

I had to unlearn, unravel, and start again to find myself in my late 40s. But you don't have to wait that long.

This is me, lighting the path ahead so you don't have to walk it alone.

And to my son Levi, this is for you too, my boy.

Because one day, you may be the partner of someone going through all of this. And I want you to understand what that means – not just the symptoms, but the emotional weight it can carry. The identity shift. The confusion. The fear. The exhaustion. The unspoken sadness that can quietly live inside the woman you love, even as she's trying her hardest to hold everything together.

I want you to be the kind of man who doesn't flinch when your partner says she doesn't feel like herself. The kind who doesn't try to fix it or ignore it, but just sits with her in it, without judgement.

I want you to be the kind of man who knows that mood swings aren't weakness. That exhaustion isn't laziness. That silence isn't rejection. You won't be able to take it all away. But you can make it easier. You can listen. You can hold her. You can say, "I see you. I'm here. What do you need?"

Because being educated about menopause isn't just about hormones and hot flashes, it's about empathy. And I want you to have the emotional intelligence to love deeply and the strength to stand beside a woman in her most vulnerable season.

If you ever forget, or wonder what to do, come back to these pages. Let this book be a guide for you too.

Contents

PART 1 ~ 1
Going Up in Flames

PART 2 ~ 35
Rising From the Ashes

PART 3 ~ 65
Walking Through the Fire as a Warrior

PART 4 ~ 115
Navigating Relationships

PART 5 ~ 137
Moving into the Future with
Wisdom and Wholeness

About the Author ~ 179
Connect With Me ~ 181
Acknowledgements ~ 183
Endnotes ~ 186

PART 1

Going Up in Flames

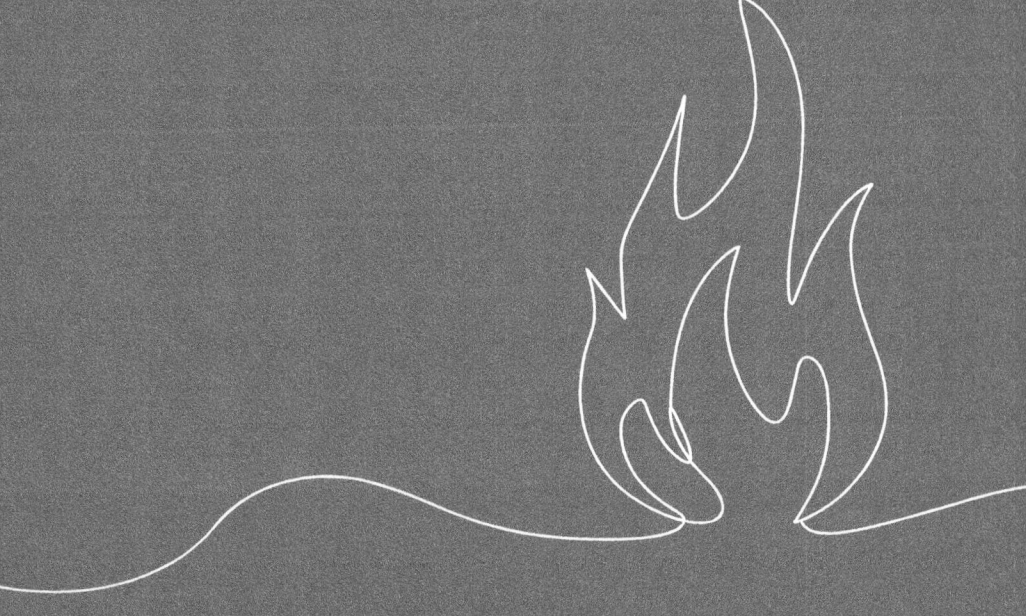

After decades of giving to others, menopause begs us to start asking: What about me?

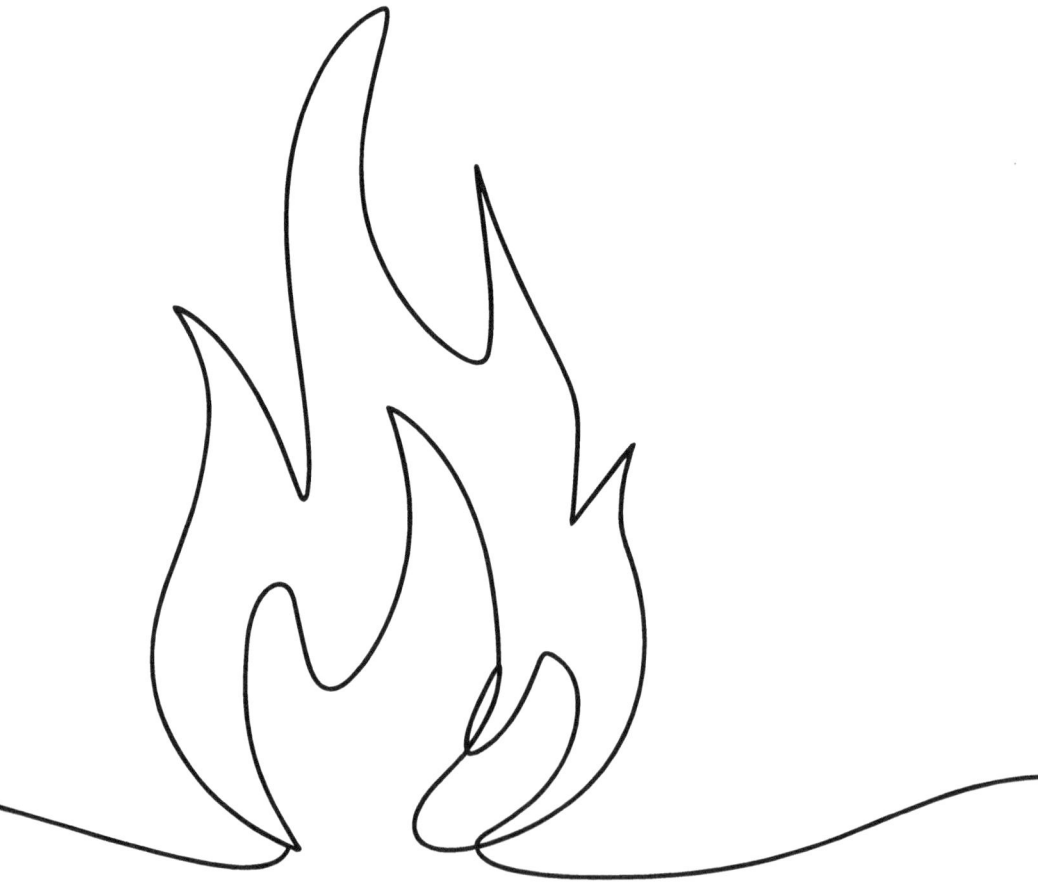

It felt like the first time I got my period. I was 10 and thought I was dying. No one had told me what was coming.

My grandparents had come over for a visit and it was a special time for me as they had brought me a glory box. While they were there, I went to the toilet and saw blood. They stayed longer than anticipated and I became more and more scared as I desperately needed Mum's attention. Once they left, I called Mum into my bedroom and told her. She explained it briefly to me before smiling and saying, "You're a woman now," while handing me a pad the size of a surfboard. I was confused and overwhelmed.

Perimenopause felt eerily similar, except now it was the *end* of being a woman. My purpose – ovulating, birthing, bleeding – was winding down. But it wasn't the gentle unwinding I imagined either. I thought I would just stop getting my period and maybe have some hot flushes, but the reality was much more complex and draining than that. It was brain fog, energy depletion, unjustified rage, sadness, a betrayal from the body, and an inability to sleep.

The result? A full-on fucking breakdown.

And So It Begins...

It started for me 3 years ago when I thought I had it all under control. I was on a roll – I'd lost 22 kilograms, my hair felt great and I felt healthy and strong. Then out of nowhere… Bam! I was shovelling churros into my mouth, my body became bloated, I gained 8 kilograms within weeks, and everything ached. I was exhausted, moody, swollen, and just… off. I felt sad and lost, but I didn't know why.

I have Hashimoto's disease, which is a thyroid condition that can cause all of the above symptoms, so I mistakenly attributed it to that and didn't think much else about it. However, during one of my routine appointments with my hormonal doctor, she flagged that it would be worth getting a blood test to determine if I was in perimenopause. The results came back a few days later, and yep it was official: my womanhood as I knew it was over. My health indicators pointed towards full-blown peri.

In the following months, I began to drink more than I ever had before at outings. I wasn't one to drink every night, but it was more binge drinking when I went out. It felt like I was celebrating something even if I didn't fully know what. Now that my four kids were older, I felt like I had a license to do whatever I wanted to, and I soon found myself getting out-of-control drunk at every party. My kids said, "What the f*ck Mum, we are the ones supposed to be getting drunk, not you."

Looking back, I think I was trying to celebrate the last of me. The 'me' I had known for so long. I was partying hard, pretending to be invincible and using alcohol as a short break from reality. The problem was, I didn't care about the aftermath. It was like I was shedding the version of myself who used to care and everything about me that no longer fit.

Meanwhile I still needed something to manage the slew of symptoms that had taken over my body (and life). My doctor suggested patches for estrogen and I felt like a walking chemist – patches for this, pills for that, cream for something else, and medication for my thyroid. I tried the patches and the cream, and maybe they helped a little with sleep, but even still I was not the same person I had been before. I then opted for the troche form, which has both estrogen and progesterone in them.

Wading Through the Fog

Brain fog is exactly what it sounds like – a fuzziness that pervades everyday thoughts and makes everything harder. And I had it bad. I was suddenly forgetting words and repeating myself constantly. It felt like my brain was filled with voices competing for space. I'd ask my husband or kids to do something and then ask again two minutes later. The worst part was that I didn't even remember saying it the first time.

My husband, Pip, sold the kids' scooters and he asked if I could put the cash in their bank accounts. I told him I could do it the next day and to put the money in an envelope in my purse. Two hours later, I was tidying up the house before bed and emptying out all the junk in my purse. I picked up the envelope and thought it was just a piece of paper and put it in the bin.

The next day, he asked, "What did you do with the envelope of money?"

I replied that it was in my bag.

He had a look and said, "No, it's not."

He looked at our security cameras and saw me put it in the

bin. Watching me, it was clear that I wasn't even registering or thinking about what I was doing.

This was unsettling for me to see. I was always so organised and switched on, but here I was throwing out an envelope of money and forgetting what I had said minutes prior. Not to mention the times I'd find the milk in the cupboard and blame Pip or the kids, before realising that it was probably me who did it.

I felt like I was going crazy. The sad thing was, so did my family.

The Double Disappearing Act of Sleep and Energy

As soon as you get pregnant, sleep becomes an elusive beast that you spend the rest of your adulthood chasing after. We go from struggling to sleep when pregnant because of the discomfort, to having a newborn and getting interrupted sleep, and then doing it all over again if you have multiple kids. You might have a few years of respite in there, but then comes the teenage stage where you're awake worrying about them or waiting to pick them up from their late nights out. You think as the kids get older that this is the time you can actually get some fucking sleep, but nope, think again because menopause has other plans.

There I was wide awake between 2 and 4am after numerous trips to the toilet, just like when I was pregnant. But this time there was no baby, you're just being punished for no reason. I walked into the door frame many times, but then I was going so often that I learnt the route and could literally do it with my eyes closed. The restlessness would get so bad that I would cave and watch a movie, you know, because I didn't have work the next day or anything! I tried so many different relaxation sounds and music to ease me back to sleep that it felt like I had a whole bloody orchestra in the room (plus my husband snoring). There were nights I just couldn't go to sleep at all, and I would only wind down at around 4am, but then only an hour later, my husband would get out of bed to head to work and any slight sound or movement would wake me up. It got to the point where he would grab his clothes off the chair where he laid them out the night before and leave the room with no lights so I didn't wake up. He would go downstairs to finish getting ready for work so he didn't wake me. Even so, my own dreaded alarm would go off at 6am. Sometimes he would sleep on the couch to try and help, but it would make no difference for me.

> **On the occasional nights where I would sleep right through, I'd wake up in absolute disbelief and ask myself, "Wow did that actually happen?"**

Other nights, I'd wake up at 11:30 and not get back to sleep until 2am before waking up again at 4am. It got to a point where I became fussy with what I wore to bed. I couldn't have anything around my neck as it felt like I was choking, and I could only wear cotton singlets because anything other than that was too hot. It was like the children's song, "Put your left foot out, put your left foot in, put your left foot out and you shake it all around." It was literally my version of the 'Hokey Pokey', but if that wasn't working and I was still too hot, I would have to go out to my balcony and sit out there until I cooled down. My balcony was my saviour, as I just needed to sit outside, let the cool air hit my face to regulate my temperature, and then head back to bed.

By lunchtime, my eyelids would get so heavy I could barely stay upright, but shit still needed to get done regardless. I would start counting the hours where I could fit in a few extra hours of sleep since I was missing so much at night, and more importantly, I was missing that deep, restorative sleep. Sometimes I'd sneak in a nap just to survive the second half of my day, but the exhaustion permeated my overall mood and energy levels. I felt like I had to be careful where I invested my energy, and if I used too much I would be in trouble. If we had an outing on a Saturday night, I wouldn't get out of bed literally all day on Sunday, going in and out of sleep. And having an autoimmune disease made me feel even more exhausted.

How did I cope with this given I have a husband and four kids and am an entrepreneur of multiple businesses? Not well. It was hard. My husband wanted to go for a walk on Sunday mornings and I'd have to constantly decline and tell him to go alone. I needed to sleep and my best sleep was always in the morning. While all this was all happening, I also got a sore shoulder that restricted movement. After a lot of research, it said it was completely common, but it would keep me up at night and it didn't matter how much magnesium or pain meds I took, it was still there.

As Pip became more involved in what was actually happening to my body and how it all worked, he would keep trying to get me out for the Sunday walk. But my mind would not concede and I just didn't want to connect with my body. All he ever wanted was to walk the coast as a couple, but I became a recluse – staying home where I felt safe.

Without even factoring in the sleep issues, the fatigue was unbearable in itself and it led to a decrease in both my mental and emotional energy. The small talk and the fake smiles disappeared quickly, and I started conserving myself. Only speaking when it mattered, trying to say 'no' a lot more, listening to my body. If I was tired, I rested. If I needed to nap, I would come in from the studio and sleep on the couch. And the sleep that would hit was *deep* – like blackout, where-am-I kind of sleep.

That had never been an option before. There was always something else to do – dinner, laundry, groceries. Now? I had no choice. It was either give myself what I needed or run myself into the ground. There was no pushing through to just make it work anymore. And what was my mood like? Well let's just say, no sleep meant I was super frustrated and would have to pre warn my family to put them on alert.

> Your body is talking. Menopause
> is your chance to finally listen.

The worst greeting someone could give me was, "How are you? You look tired." Well yes Karen, thanks for the reminder, I was tired. Tired of everything. Even things I used to enjoy – like preparing thoughtful gifts – started slipping. If I didn't have time, it was money in a card and done. I eventually pulled away from socialising altogether. I didn't have the energy to make conversations, or if I went I would start yawning because I wanted my couch. The TV and the phone couldn't talk back to me and I didn't have to try – my brain didn't have to work.

Burning Through the Heat and Rage

And let's not forget about the all-consuming rage. This isn't the normal kind of anger, but it's the one where you feel like screaming because it's building up inside of you and it becomes almost claustrophobic in its intensity. You feel fucking crazy because it's not justified emotions. It's the way someone chewed. The TV volume was too loud. The overpowering perfume. A harmless joke thrown at me but landing like a grenade. Everything grated on me. I wanted peace, and I craved silence more than anything.

It reminds me of a time when we were all sitting in my mum and dad's lounge room and my dad said something that prompted my mum to have this angry attack at him. Not only did we sit there dumbfounded and with our mouths wide open, but I think she even shocked herself with how aggressive her outburst was and how loud she screamed at him.

I called out and said, "Mum, what was that for?" At the time, I had no idea what was going on, but now that I'm going through this and having similar experiences, I wish I had been educated more so I could have responded with "Are you okay, Mum? What can I do?" Now, I wonder if this was her cry for help? Or how she tried to cope with what is now happening to me? I'd just had my first baby at this time, so I was experiencing my fluctuating hormones or at least trying to get them back to where they were, and then there was my mum at the other end trying to deal with her own changes. The only difference was that she never spoke about it.

The way she dealt with it was the easiest. She would lash out at my dad to get it off her chest and then go spend her quiet time in the garden away from everyone. She would use my dad as a verbal punching bag, with some days worse than others. Okay, he could be annoying, but some days her reactions were almost a cry for help but she wasn't heard. Her garden was her escape. She would disappear for hours and she wanted to be left alone. It was her place of peace.

This type of rage wasn't just hormonal though. It wasn't just the low estrogen or high cortisol, it was everything that had been silenced or suppressed for decades. All of a sudden, you erupt like a volcano and it's forcibly brought to the surface. It was the manifestation of resentment. Resentment for carrying the invisible load, the exhaustion of being the emotional anchor for everyone else, the pain of being overlooked, dismissed or interrupted, and the grief of a body that doesn't feel familiar or like you anymore.

It felt so out of the ordinary because we have always been taught to be agreeable, keep the peace, and to put other people's emotions before ours. Then we say what we feel deep within us and we are dismissed. Someone puts the lid back on the boiling pot and there comes a point where we go, "No, I'm not doing this anymore."

So when the rage arrives, we panic. We of course doubt ourselves and we question. *What just happened? What happened to Mum? What has gotten into you?* Not sure, but all the buried rage fuelled with bitterness, resentment and depression was surfacing. It was a sign to say that we have tolerated the same shit for so long and then we purge from deep inside. Once you have lit your fire, it's as if we are burning away the old self and when the fire goes out, it's like we no longer apologise for no reason at all – we choose peace and it refines us into the women we are supposed to be.

> Hot flashes? No – just a reminder that I'm on fire.

Joining this rage was of course the heat. Oh god, the heat. I've had thyroid issues for over 18 years, so I'm used to being cold, but when menopause started, I was sweating hot and I craved the ocean. Like everyday, I had to go for a swim. On one Sunday morning, I hadn't slept all night and I was just lying there boiling hot. I told my husband that I needed to go to the beach for a swim. He was as shocked as I was about this because it was out of character for me, but he was like, "Okay, let's go." Normally, I'm one of those people who slowly enter the water, step by step until I get comfortable to the temperature. But on this morning, I just ran and dived straight in. I felt cooled down immediately; it was like putting out the fire and I stopped sizzling. My husband stood there looking at me gobsmacked and thinking, *who are you?*

That particular summer, the ocean dip became my therapy.

All I needed was the beach: the therapeutic sound of the waves, my book, and dipping in and out of the water. I even met other local ladies who were doing the same thing.

Betrayed By the Body Once Again

Menopause feels like one final fat betrayal from your body, just like puberty or pregnancy. My boobs hurt, my belly was bloated, my body screamed for sugar. My skin itched so badly I'd scratch until I bled. I looked in the mirror and didn't recognise myself. My neck became excessively wrinkly and I was very self conscious of it. I had just completed a videoshoot for my brand and I was excited to show my sister when it went up on socials. Her response was that she couldn't take her focus off my neck. *Boom.* In came a hard hit to my self-esteem.

I didn't want to dress up. When I went shopping for an outfit for an occasion, nothing appealed to me, nor did I look good in anything I tried on. I didn't want to go out. I just wanted to hide. My senses changed too. Smells I used to tolerate – like steak and chicken – repulsed me. Perfumes I once loved gave me allergy-like symptoms, or if someone had too much on, it would smack me in the face. Dust set me off. Even my vision went. One day I could see perfectly, and the next I couldn't read a label.

It was in the early stages of peri that I first noticed something was off with my eyesight. Words in books weren't as clear anymore and I'd find myself holding the page further away, squinting, blaming the light. Then the street signs started to blur a little too and I became more cautious driving. Not terrified, just… unsure. It was like I didn't fully trust myself being behind the wheel anymore.

And that's when it hit me – I've turned into those old

drivers I used to beep at on the freeway. You know, the ones I'd impatiently overtake thinking, *Come on, love, speed up!* Now I completely get it. That feeling of hesitating, second-guessing, and not having full confidence. I have a whole new level of respect for them now.

So, I booked an appointment at my local optometrist. We talked about lenses, frames, all the usual stuff, and I waited for the call to come in and pick them up. When they finally called, I felt nervous, as this was the 'upgrade' I didn't want to face.

The moment I tried them on, I looked in the mirror and felt sick. I wanted to cry. Or scream. Or just walk straight out. The lenses were thick, like glass bottle thick, and made my eyes look huge. I couldn't believe it. I actually remembered a movie scene with a lady wearing similar glasses and I kept seeing her in the mirror.

I just stood there, staring at myself, completely mortified. *Nope.* I'm not wearing these. It was like my reflection had aged overnight. Surely they could upgrade the prescription without them looking like magnified lenses.

When one of my clients came in, we spoke about my story and she suggested I see her optometrist. So I did. This new optometrist was really good, with nearly an hour of proper testing. I showed him the glasses and said, "I'm not going to be seen dead in these."

He laughed and said, "Don't worry, we can fix that."

And he did.

When I put on the new pair, I could see properly again

and they looked normal. The relief was huge. But it wasn't just about seeing clearer, it was facing what menopause was quietly showing me.

It's funny how no one tells you how emotional it can feel when parts of your body start changing. It's not just your mind or hormones; it's everything. Your eyes, your skin, your energy. I wasn't mourning vanity – I was mourning the old version of me that could read a street sign without a second thought. Menopause brings all of it to the surface.

These days, I think of those glasses as more than just lenses; they're a symbol of how I'm learning to see myself again. Menopause has this way of stripping you back, forcing you to refocus. It's uncomfortable, but it's also grounding.

Maybe the change in my eyesight wasn't just physical, maybe it was about seeing life with new clarity. A softer, slower kind. The kind that says, you're still you – just a little more in focus. They have become my statement in photoshoots, where they finish my look and it's me, the new me.

However, one thing I still haven't come to terms with is the changes to my hair. My hair, which as a hairdresser is obviously my pride and joy, had also started thinning. I used to wash my hair once a week and be able to wake up and re-blow-dry my hair, but that's definitely not the case anymore. I've always had thick curly hair and it was never greasy, but now I have such greasy roots that my beloved blow-dry wouldn't last. I'd also have the frizz created overnight near the nape of my neck, so I had to wash my hair like three or so times a week to remove the grease. But as peri continued, it then began to feel a lot more frizzy, fine and limp and it also started falling out strand by strand. *Stunning.* I would even scare myself looking in the mirror with how wild it would look. I looked like a bird that had been electrocuted. When I blowdried my hair, it became so thin you could see right through it. My mum even noticed and became worried and made me a rosemary concoction she had seen on socials.

I also couldn't handle the sensation of it around my neck anymore, so it would always go up in a bun quicker than normal. I tried different products and nothing was working. If I went too hydrating, it made my hair even more limp, but if I opted for products designed for fine hair or volume, it made it too dry. If I used a serum, it couldn't be too much or too heavy as it would make my hair greasier quicker. I couldn't win.

One bonus of losing my hair was that when I went to shave my legs, there was just pathetic patches of hair. Three or so weeks would go by and all I've got is a few strands to shave. And let's say moisturiser was my best friend; I couldn't get enough of it. My body was so dry and my legs were super scaly like a fish. I would go for a massage and the poor masseuse would have to keep stopping to add more oil to my back as it would just get sucked in. She would say, "Ohhh, you are so dry." Yep, I was so aware. Sorry that I have literally wasted your whole bottle of oil. Did I feel super embarrassed? Sure did. No matter how much moisturiser I put on my face, it never felt hydrated. My whole body was dry – and I mean my whole body. My skin, my mouth, my eyes, it was like I had no water when I blinked. I drank so much water but I still felt dehydrated.

I ended up getting some hydration drops to put in my water but couldn't use it too much as it would send me straight to the toilet. I then tried Celtic salt in my water, and now I drink electrolytes everyday.

After the ordeal of showering, I'd drag my feet to find something to wear, and even that became impossible. I felt swollen. Did I have the urge to put something on and feel good about myself? Nope, I'd just put something on, slick that shitty hair back, force half a smile and begin my day. I didn't dare look in the mirror. I felt like a balloon ready to burst, like that feeling when you bend over to put your socks on and everything feels like a struggle. Not to mention the kangaroo pouch that grew overnight around my belly. *Where the fuck did this come from?* It arrived like an uninvited guest and didn't leave.

I would also look at my hands and see my fingers were changing. Every time I got my nails done, the nail beds looked slightly crooked on both my fingers and toes. I would always ask the nail technician if they could straighten up the nail or square it up, but it wasn't them, it was how my toes were beginning to shape as well as my fingers – swaying more to the right.

To top it off, the left side of my hip area and my glutes were tight, and I would limp when I would go from sitting to standing. I would wake up and feel like my grandma and walk how she would, slightly dipped to one side, a few cracks at the knees and the sorest feet ever. For some reason my left leg would swell at times, and it was always around my knee. It didn't matter if I went for a massage, did physio or had injections to help with the pain, it felt like nothing worked. Even on the rare occasion that it did, it would only be for a few days or a couple of weeks and then the pain would start again. Theracurmin tablets became my best friend to reduce inflammation.

It didn't help that I had stopped exercising when the symptoms started, so I didn't have that energy release or endorphin source. I used to be quite active, alternating between the gym, yoga and walking, but soon I was too tired and sore to do anything. It was the first thing to be sacrificed in lieu of more sleep and an attempt to maintain energy levels; however, it probably didn't help and it was a vicious cycle that I couldn't get out of.

This inflammation also affected my feet, and all of a sudden I couldn't wear heels anymore. Something that honestly was kind of devastating for me. When I was younger and I'd go out clubbing on the weekends, no heel was ever too high. The higher, the better. Chunky, strappy, pointed, wild – heels were my thing. My guilty pleasure. My fashion fetish.

And sore feet? Hell no. I could jump from bar to club, dance all night, walk to the local kebab joint at 2am, hail down a taxi like a woman on a mission and never once complain about foot pain. That's just how it was. Heels were part of the uniform.

I remember asking my mum one day, "Why don't you wear heels anymore?"

Completely unaware. Clueless. I didn't know what menopause really was, as it never occurred to me. She looked at me and said: "Don't you think I'd love to? Of course I would. But I can't. My feet hurt too much."

I urged her, "Come on Mum, just try…"

And she would, every now and then, especially if we were going somewhere nice. But she'd always end up in pain. I understood, but I didn't fully get it. Not until it happened to me…

It was the races. I'd just started peri and I had bought these new heels that were gorgeous. But 2 hours in and it was like my feet had been shoved into medieval torture devices. The fat on the top of my feet had imprinted into the lines of the shoes so deep, they looked bruised. I couldn't even get them off. Pip had to piggyback me to the Uber.

No joke, the heels went straight into the bin on the way out. I got home, dumped my feet in ice, and almost cried. That was the moment everything changed.

From then on, it was leather heels only. No cheap, stiff pairs. A thicker heel for support. Comfort over cuteness. It has just gotten worse over the years too, so now I'm down to the lowest heel possible, just enough to make the outfit work. How sad is that? I used to swear I'd never change my shoes halfway through an event. But now I'll host an event, greet everyone, take photos, say my speech and off they come. Straight into flats or slides before dessert has even been served. I'd carry an extra bag with me just for my second pair of shoes.

With all this change, it just felt like a giant slap in the face. I had spent all these years building an identity and a self-care routine and now all of a sudden it had been stripped from me and it seemed like there was nothing I could do to control it. I was never confident in my looks and body growing up, and the changes through peri felt the same as the transition from being a young girl to a teen and then a teen to a young adult. It was those same thoughts and questioning.

Misunderstood, Moody and Just Sad

Let's not forget about our emotions. I went and watched *Tina the Musical* and I cried and cried. It was a beautiful musical but the storyline made me sob. I was more sensitive, and I took everything to heart. The kids would say, "Mum, it's not that deep", but I'd have taken it in a deep, sensitive way. Everything hit me harder, especially thinking about how strong of a woman Tina was and the story of her life, her strength and her courage. She didn't give up.

I tried to be strong, so when it finally came out, it poured out and I started to question my self worth. *Who are you? What's your purpose? Does anyone understand?* People would say, "Oh, but it's just menopause. It can't be that bad", but I just wanted to be heard.

In the early days, I felt lost and would drive in my car around the streets, wanting to be on my own. I'd just sit in the car and watch the sunset. I'd cry at movies or anything that upset me – I felt fragile.

It was at this time that I discovered Rufus Du Sol. They were my go-to artist every time I got in the car. Even my kids were like, "Who are they?" A year on, they came to Perth and I had to go see them. There's this particular song called 'Underwater' that I would sit and listen to on repeat and tears would literally stream down my face. It described exactly how I felt at the time. Stuck, underwater, and like I needed some space. I felt like I was drowning.

My kids were getting older and so I had to deal with not feeling needed as much as I used to, as they were their own people now. I'd constantly juggle trying to check in on all four kids and take an interest in what's going on, but I would forget at times or not be fully present. And then I had Pip, who had his own business and came home just as exhausted, but it's like, "Hey what about me? Can someone listen and hear me?" Everyone had their own life and problems, and I didn't want to burden my family or friends, so I was trying to balance it all and it was just getting too much. I didn't have the mental or physical capacity.

It seemed everything ended in an argument and no one could see my point of view when I did try to express how I was feeling. One afternoon, I had an argument with my younger two, Caprice and Armani, and it was two against one. I felt like I was losing the battle. My mum happened to come by and the argument continued, and she was like to the girls, "This isn't your mum's fault."

Armani was like, "Yeah well, when is this menopause going to end?"

My mum and I looked at one another and then she

replied, "Nice one girls, I have some news for you. It's here to stay for a while."

The next thing I got asked was, "How come other mums don't talk about menopause?" Since that comment, I kept it more to myself. I said less, but my emotions said more. I feel it's unfair that mothers, and women in general, are going through a change while their teens are also going through their own hormonal journey. When I would go through a rage or a mood swing, it was all symptoms minus being on a period, so this is how I explained it to the girls. I had to listen and deal with their hormonal journey and it was only fair that they could be more sympathetic with me instead of against me. I just felt life wasn't fair… When you don't feel like yourself but you have to still show up as a mother when your teens need you the most. It was all about them: their journey and the advice they needed. Meanwhile, I was at my most vulnerable and the lowest time of my life.

Everything frustrated me. The clinking of the bowl, the extra loud chewing, the dishes left in the sink. I was constantly sad and angry. I stopped listening to music and I even had to beg my husband to take our dog to work with him because he barked a lot and all of a sudden the sound pierced through my nerves like a jackhammer. Even in silence, I sometimes heard the phantom barking echoing in my brain.

I became even more aware when I would speak to friends or clients that I sounded sad and negative. I was angry at everything. I would hold onto more negative thinking rather than try to turn it into a positive like I used to do. This didn't help me being a mother when I was supposed to be a role model guiding them into their worlds of thinking more positively and not focusing on the negative. But how was I supposed to do this when all I felt was angry at the world and angry at myself? I felt I was deep in a hole.

It's like I had lost myself. How could I love more when I had stopped loving myself? How could I give more when I felt so tired and fatigued? No one understood, no one got it – my body had no more fuel in the tank to keep chugging along. I was just fucking tired. I would talk to myself to try to make myself believe that I wasn't tired and respond with, "Yes I am good", but my face said it all, especially the bags under my eyes.

Deep thoughts start to enter when your brain is fogged up like this. *What would it be like if I disappeared? Would it be easier on everyone not to deal with me? Why did I feel I was going crazy, like batshit crazy?*

My family and friends would bypass me and go straight to Pip to have a conversation, and I would feel envy bubble to the surface, as he was always the one who was praised. On the outside looking in, they saw a strong Wendy, but on the inside, I was broken, alone and invisible. My brain was constantly full and racing with thoughts like: *Did I do that, I need to go pick that up, what formula did I use on my client?* The thoughts were unstoppable. They would float in my mind and then I would be talking myself out of it.

> Menopause is messy, moody and
> maddening, but you are not alone.

I've never liked the word depressed or depression. If I spoke with my husband, I would describe it as I feel sad – like REAL sad. Or if it got too much, I would be like I need you! But as a man, it was hard for him to truly understand. When I got into a really heavy, lonely space, the words would come out: "I just need you." *But how did I need him?* I didn't know and neither did he.

All I knew was that I wasn't coping mentally and physically. Did I want him around? Yes, but also no because it irritated me at the same time, so I didn't know what I wanted. His response was, "What is wrong with you? Why are you yelling? It's not a big deal." But everything felt like it was. I had to get my voice heard and my point of view was right the way I saw it. I couldn't answer him because I didn't know. It was like, "I think you need to help me see and deal with all this because I can't do this on my own."

> Validation for what we are going through
> can make the difference between feeling
> crazy and feeling understood.

Pip took it upon himself to read a bit more, listen to podcasts and try and educate himself through it. But when it comes down to it, what does "I understand" really mean? How can they possibly understand? At times, I would lean more on my eldest for support, but then at the same time, I didn't want to burden her. She had her own issues and I felt it was unfair to bog her down (or anyone else for that matter) with mine. I guess the answers had to come from me, or I had to become the answer.

The Breaking Point

After 3 years of debilitating symptoms that had worn me down to a shell of myself, I finally snapped.

Sundays used to be my productive day where I'd get the shopping, washing and food prepping done, but now I could barely get myself out of bed and I didn't even care. The fridge was empty? So what. The washing basket was overflowing? Oh well. It's like you all of a sudden reach a limit and think, *why is this all left to me? Or why is it expected of me?* When it became more frequent, my husband started to get food shopping on the way home, and if I didn't feel like cooking dinner, I just simply didn't. For the first time ever, I wasn't running the household like a military unit. I had no energy and even less interest.

I started asking myself, *is this all I've been to my family this whole time? The cleaner, the chef, the shopping bitch, the schedule keeper, the crisis manager?* It's only now that I've finally stopped and asked, *where have I gone?* As an actual person, not just a mum and wife. I realised I had mimicked my grandma and mum, as they were both hard workers and taught me to be the cleaner and cook and to agree with my husband to keep him happy. They didn't have much of a voice in the family, so that's what I had taken on as being the right thing. But it wasn't natural to me. I was more independent and I don't like being told what to do. Now this was all coming to the surface. All the resentment. I used to stop mid-client to throw on a load of washing or come in from the salon quickly to stir a pot on the stove. But no one noticed. I would watch everyone come home and even though I'd been at work all day too, everyone else got to go rest on their phones or lay down but all I heard was, "What's for dinner?"

I felt like no one wanted me. Not my husband. Not my kids. Comments would fly, casually cruel, like, "OMG, Dad, why did you even marry her?"

Let me tell you how that feels: it farking hurts. After everything I've done and continue to do, I was left questioning: *Why am I even here?* I reached a point where I didn't want to argue anymore. I didn't want to be stirred or tested. I just wanted to be left alone. Walk away. Let me be. I remember one night, mid-argument with my husband, he threw a line so sharp I could feel my whole body go cold: "If I knew you now, I don't think I'd marry you." And just when I thought it couldn't get worse, he followed it up with, "You're not the girl I married."

No shit, Sherlock. Of course I'm not the same girl. I was young, naive, a peace-maker, and said yes to everything. Since then, I've become a woman who's birthed four humans, built a business, carried a household, and still kept going.

It got to the point where I finally thought, *fuck it. I'm done.*

> **Menopause gave me permission to stop apologising and start prioritising.**

I went on strike. For the first time in my life, I let the house go. Fingerprints on benches. Crumbs on the floor. Dirty clothes still in baskets. Did it bother me? God, yes. But I forced myself to look away. To let it slide. To not care. But not caring felt weird. Wrong. Almost rebellious. If only everyone could contribute, but instead it was expected that I would do it all.

"Mum, did you iron my shirt?"

"Nope."

"Why not?"

"I forgot."

"That's rude."

But then this sent everyone into a frantic turmoil. *What's wrong with Mum? Why is she so angry?* I didn't know, but everything bothered the shit out of me and I just stopped caring. I had always been the one who showed love by doing. The loving, caring mum who always made their school lunches, washed their clothes or emptied the dishwasher. I did as I was asked, tried to please everyone, not upset them and be supportive. But

I was burning out. I started to feel selfish about feeling selfish, but I also didn't care.

I was erupting like a volcano. Loudly. Unapologetically. Not because I wanted to hurt anyone, but because I needed to be heard. I needed them to know that Mum was still here, buried under the weight of expectations, hot flashes, aching joints, and sleepless nights. And if they wanted her to stick around, she needed a little less pressure and a lot more space to breathe. To be asked, "How are you, Mum? What can I do to make it easier for you?" It's the simplest things that help take the pressure off me – the times when they think for themselves or take some initiative.

It was Christmas that finally broke me. It's my favourite time of year. I love the lights, the traditions, the food, the joy of giving. But with perimenopause creeping in and work already demanding so much, I was running on empty. I was tired, overwhelmed, stretched thin by the pressure of organising gifts, food and plans for everyone else. When the adrenaline of 'go, go, go' finally stopped, I crashed hard. And that Christmas, the crash was brutal.

I unwrapped my gifts. From my husband, I got a MacBook that had been bought two days before Christmas. We needed it for the business because the old computer was crashing, and it could be claimed on tax. It was a practical, logical and sensible gift – not to mention very expensive. But in that moment, it felt a bit like getting a vacuum cleaner for your birthday – useful and necessary, but not a gift chosen with me in mind.

From my children came the apron they'd seen trending on TikTok and a scissor pouch. In 30 years as a hairdresser, I've never worn a scissor pouch. I've avoided them for a reason. Yet here I was, opening gifts that screamed: tools for work, tools for serving, tools for everyone else.

I remember sitting there trying to be grateful, but the tears started before I even knew how to stop them. Not because I was ungrateful, not because I was spoiled, but because, in that moment, I felt reduced to the roles I filled, not the woman I was. I sobbed and sobbed. My words spilled out between tears: "Is this my worth to you? Is this how you see me?"

To me, those gifts said: "You're the worker, the organiser, the giver." Not Wendy, the woman who deserves to be surprised, delighted, and seen. But to them, it was nothing so deep. "Mum, you're being ungrateful. It's not that serious."

And just like that, my pain became the problem.

And instantly I felt alone. I wasn't seen nor heard; I was invisible to my family. And the saddest of it all was that not one of them had my back. I felt like I was left out in the cold. Growing up, I was always so supportive of my mum, no matter if she was right or wrong. But my kids weren't the same.

I was told I had ruined Christmas. That my crying had dampened the day. But what no one did was come up to me, put their arms around me, and say, "I'm sorry you feel like this. We didn't mean to upset you." They thought I had taken it too far by crying and again trying to express my thoughts only to be shut down, but to them it was so odd. I definitely must have looked like a lunatic.

I put on my sunglasses, hiding tears as we drove to my

brother's house for lunch. He asked if I was okay. "Yes, all good," I lied, because I couldn't spoil his Christmas too. But inside I wanted to curl up in a hole. I felt alone, invisible, ignored. The world around me celebrated while I sat in silence, aching with the sense that I didn't matter.

Looking back, I can see it wasn't about the laptop, or the apron, or the scissor pouch. It was about what those gifts represented: A woman who was seen for her function rather than her heart. A mother and wife who gives endlessly but longs to be seen in her own right. A soul already fragile from hormonal shifts, exhaustion and the invisible weight of menopause.

What I needed wasn't jewellery or perfume or even something expensive either. I needed recognition. Presence. Something that said, "We see you. We love you. Not for *what* you do, but for *who* you are."

If you've ever cried on Christmas Day, on your birthday, or after opening a gift that missed the mark – you're not alone.

It's not about being spoiled. It's not about being ungrateful. It's about the deep, human longing to be seen and to be known. Peri-menopause intensifies that longing. Our hormones are shifting, our energy is stretched, and our emotions are raw. The smallest thing can become the biggest wound when what we truly crave is acknowledgement and love.

So if this story feels familiar, know this: your worth is not the meals you cook or the roles you play. Your worth is in you. And sometimes, tears are the body's way of saying: I need more than practicality. I need to feel cherished.

It was around this time that Pip started to tune into what was happening. Better late than never, right? To his credit, he started becoming more present and started relieving some of the pressure. He started stepping in, without waiting for me to nag, break down or ask. He began to notice when I was drowning in the mental load and finally took initiative.

He was raised in a traditional European home where the man works and the woman stays home. The provider earns the income, and that's where his job ends. But I was like, "Mate, I also run a business and I'm raising four kids. This is mental overload." It took years for him to adjust and realise we are both business-minded people who share a family. It became clearer for Pip when he would see how these new-age dads at work were super hands-on with their newborns and toddlers, whereas I had left Pip to sleep when our children were young because I didn't feel right waking him up throughout the night when he had to be driving and handling machinery.

And throughout the whole time we had kids, if I went down, either sick, overwhelmed or burnt out, the whole ship would sink. It would take two days of chaos before Pip would step in and go, "Alright, I need to take time off work." Because the truth is, if I'm not right, nothing is. Not the kids. Not the house. Not the energy.

So when I went on strike, Pip caught on. This wasn't a moment, it was a movement. He realised, finally, that I meant business and so he began taking the lead. Asking questions like, *Who needs to be where? What needs to be done? How can I help without being asked?*

He started to see that family life needs to be shared, not assigned. That it takes a team effort to keep this machine running. Don't get me wrong – Pip's always tried in his own way, but now, he truly shows up. He started noticing when I was tired, when something hurts, when I need space and he goes into full action mode without waiting for a signal.

He's grown with me. Evolved. And ripened beautifully with age (thank God). So no, this isn't about tearing him down. It's about showing the journey. The fight. The raw truth behind so many households. And it's about saying to every woman out there:

You're not alone.

You're not a fool.

And you have every right to be the woman you've become.

PART 2

Rising From the Ashes

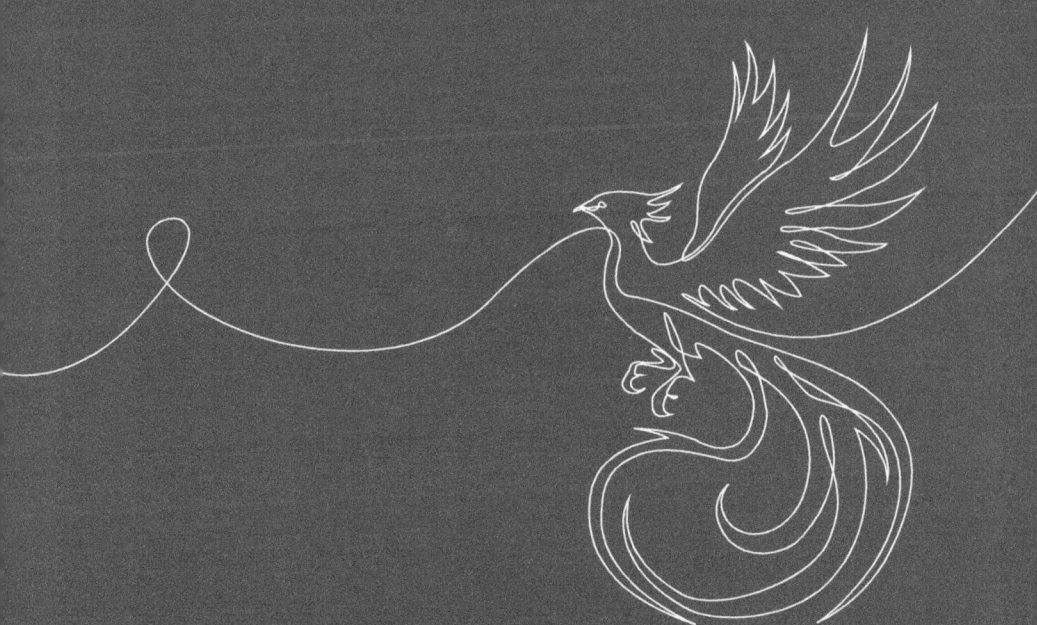

Once the fire settles and the ashes cool, a stronger, wiser and zero-tolerance-for-bullshit version of you emerges.

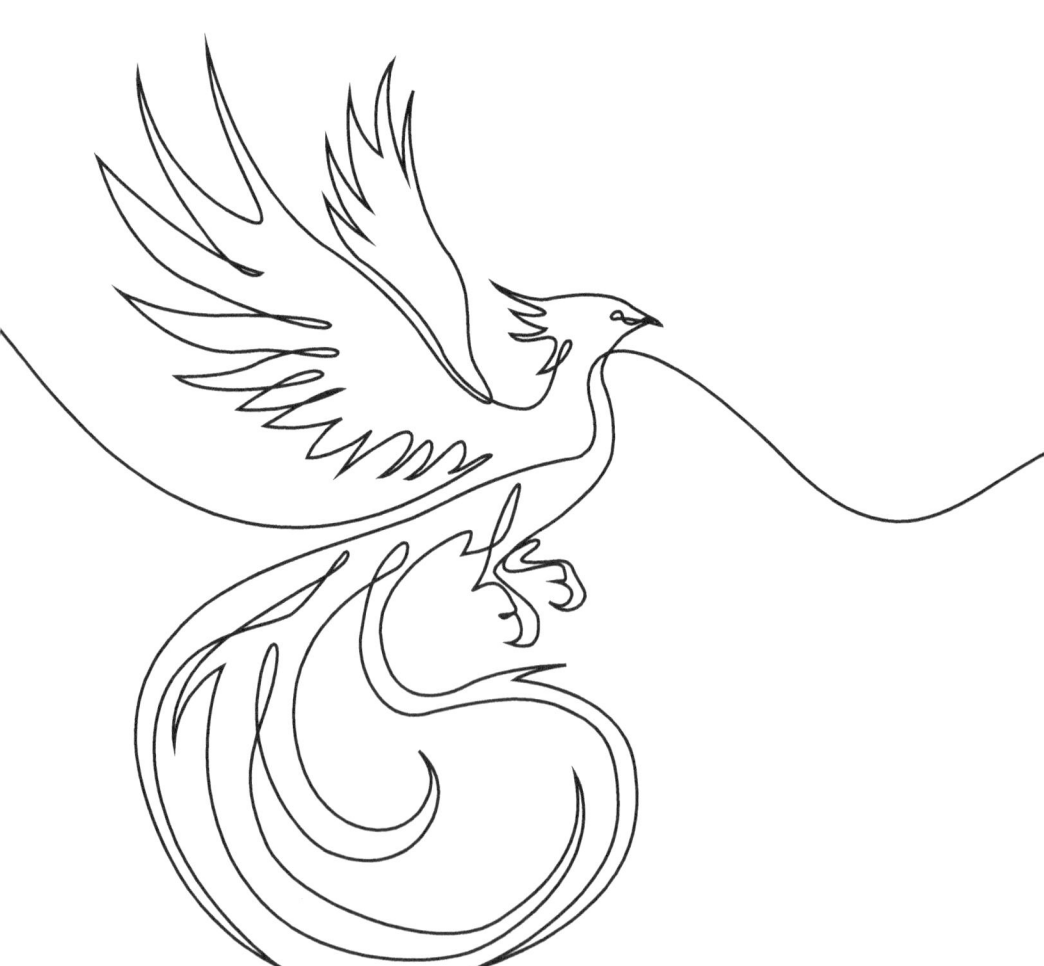

We're taught menopause means decline. That we're less desirable, less fertile, less relevant. But maybe it was just stripping us bare. Maybe it was pulling off everything that was never really ours to carry in the first place. The pressure to be liked. To be pleasant. To say yes. To smile through pain. Perimenopause burns all of that down. And in the ashes, we begin to show up in a different way. Not quieter – but more honest.

We speak when we want to. We sit in rooms and don't shrink. We stop performing. Our buried needs and dreams and grief come rising up, demanding to be acknowledged. We stop being the "good girl", or the go-getter everyone is expecting us to be, or the all-knowing guru who gets asked all the questions. But with this comes the question: *Who am I now?* Not as a mother. Not as a wife. Not as a business owner. But as *me*.

And here was what I had come to believe: this wasn't a crisis. This was a second coming of age. We aren't invisible. We're undeniable. There are still tears. There is still exhaustion. But underneath it all, there is power. There is clarity. There is *truth*.

You are not losing yourself.

You are finally meeting *her*.

Putting the Pieces Back Together

Not long after I went on strike, I found myself in a hole so dark and so heavy that I couldn't see a way out. It wasn't just sadness – it was an emptiness that consumed me from the inside out. A place where the thoughts in my head no longer felt like mine, and the silence around me was deafening.

It was lonely. Terrifying. I truly believed I was no longer needed – not by myself, not by my husband, not even by my children. My sense of worth had completely vanished. I didn't just feel invisible; I felt like I no longer existed. And yes, I thought about death. And that thought scared the shit out of me.

But perhaps the most painful part was feeling like no one understood. I was surrounded by people, yet completely alone. When I tried to speak, my pain was dismissed. "It's not that deep" or "It's just menopause, can't be that bad" – these words cut when you're barely holding on. So, I learned to brush it all aside, to keep moving, to survive. On the outside, I was functioning, but inside I felt like a ghost. Like I was living in someone else's life. Zombified. Exhausted. Disconnected from everything, including myself.

I was also dealing with a grieving process of sorts, where you grieve the loss of the younger you, your fertility, and the body you no longer recognise. But what happens when that internal grief is met with real world loss?

It was right at this time that we lost my grandmother – my baba. We said our final goodbyes a few days before Christmas, but the strong woman she was, she wasn't ready to let go. To have seen her get so thin and fragile broke my heart. I came home from Sydney on Australia Day and called Mum to see how she was. Mum said not good. I remember saying, "Why is God so cruel? Why hasn't He taken her to rest yet? Why is she still suffering?" As much as we all wanted her here with us, her body and soul needed to rest. I felt awful saying what I said but I couldn't understand why she put up a fight for so long when she was in pain.

She passed away at 8pm that night. It was like I was heard by the big man upstairs, asking kindly to take her to be reunited with my grandfather and to finally be rested with peace.

She was more than just my baba – she was my calm, my grounding, my escape from noise. I could visit her and sit holding her hand, whether we spoke or whether we sat in silence. I loved visiting her at her home, surrounded by her biggest asset and love, her garden. When I would visit, she would sit on her verandah and we would chat for hours sharing stories. I will always treasure these moments.

And then she was gone.

And I haven't been able to separate the grief of losing her from the grief of losing myself. The version of me who used to bounce back. The one who used to laugh more easily and not be so sensitive. Or the one who could cry and recover. I can't shed my tears as easily. The tiredness sits deeper, and the world feels louder, harder and more fragile.

A few weeks after losing her, I was in the bath and my body was aching. I whispered out loud, "Baba, please give me the strength to feel better." To my surprise, the lights in the bathroom flickered three times and I smiled. I knew she'd heard me. I know she is still with me, but I miss her.

And what I have come to realise is that menopause and loss

don't take turns, they overlap, they tangle and they rise together. They sharpen and deepen the ache of one another, and yet both are calling you to surrender. To feel, to let go of who and what you loved, and to find the new version of yourself that is still standing.

> Grief isn't about taking from us, it brings us clarity, courage, a softened heart and a deeper presence.

And I suppose there was a reason for me starting this book after she passed, now that I look at it. Baba may not be here physically anymore, but somehow I feel her now more than I ever have. In the flicker of the light and in the strength I didn't think I had.

It was her who gave me the strength to work on myself and try to feel good about myself again. So when I woke up one day and decided I needed to move, I knew it was her telling me I needed to get moving. Not metaphorically, but physically. My mind was screaming, and I knew I had to interrupt the noise. So I did.

Taking Back Control

I found a reformer Pilates class and simply went. No expectations. Just a hope that maybe it would help.

During this first session, my gosh, I was so stiff and wobbly. I had no balance and my legs were burning in the first 5 minutes. I couldn't even straighten them all the way when I had the ropes on. There were a few ladies in the class who were maybe my mum's age, and looking at them gliding away did make me feel like an idiot for not being able to do the exercises on the easiest pulleys. I was embarrassed, but I pushed through and kept going – taking one session at a time. I soon began to realise that it was like a 50-minute healing session.

> **My thoughts would quieten and I'd tune into my body, and then when I walked out, it was with a blissfully clear head.**

After 3 months of multiple sessions per week, I was starting to feel stronger and more centred in myself. This change made me realise that there were ways I could better manage my symptoms – ways I could take control of this menopause thing instead of letting it control me.

When I was growing up, my dad would sing to me, "Anything you want, you got it." It sounds like I was the centre of his world – the little girl who could have it all. But my dad wasn't raising me to be spoiled. The message was much deeper. He was teaching me that while anything was possible, I had to work for it, earn it and value it. This lesson echoes through my life today.

So often menopause can feel like life is stripping things away like sleep, energy, focus, even the sense of self we once knew. It can feel unfair, like the rules have changed without warning. But my dad's words remind me that I am not powerless. If I want strength or confidence, I have to choose to show up myself. It's not about waiting for someone else to give me permission, it's about me claiming it through my own actions.

Remembering How to Feel Again

Despite feeling physically better from the reformer Pilates, I still felt emotionally empty. It felt like I had forgotten what it was like to love – to feel love, to give love, even to receive it. It's hard to explain, but the part of me that once craved closeness, connection and touch just shut down. I didn't want anyone near me. Not physically and not emotionally. Sadness and anger had taken over. The version of me that once loved deeply had faded, and in its place was someone numb – tired, disconnected, lost. I had no desire to go out with friends and socialise; my ideal outing was the couch. Loving myself felt like a distant memory. I didn't even know who I was anymore, let alone how to care for her. There were times when the dark thoughts would approach and I'd experience shortness of breath and heart palpitations. I'd have to take calming tablets and do deep breathing to control myself again. It's like a fight for who's gonna win: the mind or the body. Despite all the turmoil, somewhere deep inside, I still wanted to try to feel something again.

I was chatting with a close friend who was also in the trenches of perimenopause when she said something out loud that I had absolutely felt, but never dared to say. She looked me dead in the eye and said, "Sometimes I just want to be somewhere by myself. No husband. No kids. Just me." And my whole body exhaled.

Because I had thought about it too. Many times. I had imagined what it would be like to disappear for a few days, a week, longer maybe. No responsibilities, no one asking me what's for dinner, no one needing anything. Just space. Just quiet. Just me. But how do you explain that to your husband or your kids without it sounding like rejection? Because here's what happens: you express the tiniest version of this truth – this need – and the first thing your partner asks is: "What did I do wrong? Why wouldn't you want me to come with you?"

I get it. I truly do. From the outside, it sounds like pushing them away. And that hurts. It feels personal. It triggers fear, resentment, even guilt. But the truth is, it's not about them. It's about survival. It's about self-preservation. It's about needing a moment where you don't have to be 'on' for anyone else and can just be a human with nothing but your own thoughts. And in those moments, the fantasy of escaping creeps in.

Not forever and not to punish anyone, but just to breathe again. To feel the ground under my feet without the weight of everything I carry.

This brings me to something harder to explain, but I know some of you will get it.

You know that feeling – when you want to love, to feel not just touch or routine intimacy, but that connection. The kind that lights you up from the inside, that fluttery sensation in your chest, like when you first met your partner. The butterflies. The spark. The electricity. But now I just want to feel him again, genuinely. Not just with my body, but with my soul. I know he's my person. I know we were meant to do life together. But somewhere in the chaos of motherhood, the overwhelm of responsibilities and the hormonal rewiring of menopause, something shut off. A light switch flicked off. And I find myself asking: *Where did that woman go? The one who felt everything so deeply.*

Now it's like I want him around, but not too close. I want to connect, but I also want space. I want to open up, but then I feel guilty when I can't. So I say, "I'm sorry" over and over, for not being able to show love the way I used to. But the truth is, it's still there. Buried. Raw. Waiting. It's not that I don't love him, I just need to reconnect with myself first before I can fully connect with him again. I get more connection from a healthy conversation, as talking and connecting like this makes me happy because I am being heard.

So with all this weighing me down, I signed up for a weekend sound healing retreat without overthinking it. I didn't know exactly what I was looking for, but I just knew I needed space because it was at a time when I wasn't seeing eye-to-eye with anyone in my family. I needed silence and peace, and fuck it, I'd never done anything like this before. And I'm so grateful I listened to that little nudge inside me and made the decision to just go do it. I didn't know what to expect, but I did know that it could go hand-in-hand with what was going on for me. I had attended a few of the host's sound healing classes locally and I'd loved it. It took me to a whole new place while being on a mat wrapped in a blanket.

I was scared to tell the kids and Pip what I was doing, as I was worried what their reactions would be, but they were all positive and like, "Yes Mum, you deserve some time out, you should go." That was reassuring for me.

So Friday morning arrived, I went off to Pilates and did some last minute errand drops before coming home to pack my bags. Then I jumped in the car for the 3-hour drive, blaring Madonna remixes with the sun roof open and the windows down, just enjoying the drive. I felt excited but anxious and didn't know what to expect. When I arrived, I was in the middle of nowhere, surrounded by bushland with no reception, which didn't bother me at all as I was keen for a bit of a technology detox.

I got out of the car and the silence that surrounded me was almost deafening, like super quiet. I could only hear the trees swaying in the wind and smell fresh grass and wood burning. Once everyone had arrived, we did a meet and greet and got given a sticker with our names on it. We went around to introduce ourselves before settling in. The house was super cute. The dining area was downstairs, and there were healthy green plants everywhere and a fireplace surrounded by antique couches that looked like something my baba had in her home. There were some wooden stairs leading up to where we would be sleeping, and the rooms were set up like little dormitories, with no doors, just a curtain. I chose a bed by the window and a plant. Part of me felt like a hippy and the other felt I was on school camp.

That night we had a welcome ceremony. We went around and shared our thoughts, and it felt good to speak to a bunch of women who were non-judgemental and strangers. We did some sound healing and journalling. I love to write and always have, so it was nice to put pen to paper and write down my thoughts and how I felt. This is definitely something I took away from the weekend and tried to do more of after. We had this amazing chef come cook for us over the weekend, and it was amazing. It was all so fresh and vegetarian.

What surprised me the next morning was that we weren't allowed to talk and all had to go meet in the room to silently meditate for half an hour. I'm not one for meditation, probably because I haven't done it properly before, but once I was taught how to and actually tuned into myself, I became more at peace and journalled what came up for me.

Throughout the day, I felt angry, nervous and anxious, and I couldn't work out why I was triggered. When it came to the group session and we went around to say how we were feeling, I had to pass. I don't know if I was super relaxed or had a good cleanse, but I definitely felt heavy and like I didn't have the energy to speak. It almost felt like my mind and body were weak and drained from what I had let go of in the sound healing class. I was happy to listen, and I was glad I made that decision. Another lady in the group felt the same way, which made me feel less alone with just listening and observing rather than sharing.

I met a beautiful lady at the retreat who turned 50 while we were down there. Her stories were very similar to mine, and we pulled away to have a chat before we left. When I asked her how she felt being 50, she threw her hands up in the air and said, "Yeah, well there's not really a lot to celebrate." She felt like she couldn't be herself, and I agreed. It's almost like you want to be free and without judgement. Free to be the true version of yourself without somebody making a comment or finding a fault.

> **Over the course of that weekend, something began to shift. Slowly. Gently. Like the sun breaking through after a long, dark winter.**

The final morning, I felt a lot lighter and more at ease with myself, my brain and my body. I was happy, bubbly and was loving life. While I was packing, I felt something unexpected: warmth in my chest. A soft ache of longing. I missed my kids. Not just the idea of them, but the deep, emotional connection I had struggled to feel for so long. I've always loved my children of course, but this was different. This was *feeling* it. Truly feeling it. It was just a glimpse, but it felt so good. It had been ages since I had felt anything except anger.

And that small moment changed something in me.

Once I got back home, I started investing more in myself. I kept going to Pilates and my goal was to eventually build up to doing some weight training with a good friend of mine at her gym and get toned and fit again, but my mind and body were just not quite there yet. It will all come with time and baby steps. It's all about finding the best way I can use my energy without hitting rock bottom after.

I also branched out to other forms of self care like lymphatic drainage massages and kinesiology sessions. The massages really helped because I had a lot of fluid retention and it was just super relaxing. As for the kinesiology, I was recommended to see a lady who cleanses chakras. I went in with an open mind and didn't know what to expect. We had a chat about menopause, life, family and kids before she got me to lay on the bed. I was to hold my hand here, press here, while she was hovering over my body with her hands. Every so often, she would read me an affirmation to cleanse out trauma stored within me, and the affirmations were about letting go to feel lighter again. I was there for 3 hours, and once she was done, I got off the bed, lost my balance and couldn't believe how much lighter my mind and body felt. It was like it was emptied; it was a bizarre feeling but felt amazing. She gave me drops to take in the morning and at night and told me to remember what I am grateful for in everyday life.

Being on this rollercoaster, we can get triggered super quickly and don't stop to remember what we are grateful for. I began doing this every morning and also before bed, just so I could remember to appreciate what's around me and rewrite my mindset into something more positive.

Finding a New Purpose

The introduction of these wellness habits changed the way I showed up both in the home with my family, but also in my salon. I began to listen more closely to my clients – not just to their hair goals, but to their hearts. So many women sat in my chair carrying the same weight I once held. The anxiety. The anger. The questions. "Is this perimenopause? Why do I feel like this? Why can't I control it?" Their stories echoed my own, and often, their tears mirrored mine.

I started sharing what helped me. Whether it was taking CBD oil to help calm my nervous system, going for a lymphatic massage, or attending sound healing sessions – I offered it all, not as advice, but as lived experience. And something beautiful began to happen.

They listened and they tried it. And then when they returned for their next appointment, I'd hear: "I booked in for that massage you mentioned" or "I went and did sound healing. I cried the whole time, but I needed it."

> This is the power of connection. Of sharing. Of turning a salon chair into a safe space – a place where women can feel seen, heard and supported.

We don't have to heal alone. Healing becomes less overwhelming when we walk through it together. And for me, it's become a calling to not only offer hair and beauty, but to offer something deeper: a space for emotional nourishment and community.

This also got me thinking about what I could do to support my clients firsthand.

Soon after I started going through menopause, I could tell which of my clients were going through it too, not just by their attitude and the tough bitch "don't fark with me attitude", but also by their hair.

The Inspiration For a New Path

There was a particular time I had a new client, let's call her Natalie, crying to me on the phone. She really wanted to come see me but asked if the salon could be empty at the time because she was embarrassed about the state of her hair. I did as she requested and we had a very lengthy consultation. Her hair was falling out rapidly. It was super fine, but the roots were a little oily so she was frequently washing her hair. On top of it all, she had a natural wave that consisted of frizz. Because of these challenges, she was giving up on her appearance, had no confidence and was ready to wear a wig.

One of Natalie's main concerns was when she had gone to hairdressers in the past, no one took the time to listen and hear her out. When she got a trim, her hair would separate and you could see her scalp. She didn't like this and it made her feel uncomfortable. It was obvious she was feeling a lack of confidence and didn't feel beautiful. I could relate to this, as I struggled with my confidence and self worth throughout all these changes too.

She had also resorted to a dermatologist. I'm not fully against dermatologists and what they do with their work, but after breaking down the consultation, it was obvious that no one really took the time to listen and invest in Natalie. I suggested getting off whatever was prescribed to her by the dermatologist. I researched the product and read all the chemicals that were being put on the hair. They did not help with her hair or the condition, and this was a case where menopause had simply been overlooked when prescribing the medication.

For the actual cut, I lightly trimmed the hair to give the illusion that there was some extra volume and for her hair to bring some bounce and curls. She was forever grateful and she left with a smile on her face.

A week or so later, Natalie returned as she had an event to go to and asked if I could put her hair up and do her makeup. Natalie came to her appointment with a scrunchie sort of hair piece that she wanted to put in to make her hair look thicker and give her extra body. I'm super honest and one of my biggest pet peeves is seeing a hair piece that looks super fake and does no justice for the hair. I reassured her that I could get her hair up without using that extra hair piece. She was a bit hesitant and was like, "Are you sure you can do that?" But she gave me a chance, so I waved her hair with a small tong, let it sit to build up volume and then put it up in a textured French roll.

Her facial expressions went from being unsure to a confident smile on her face. I ticked off all the boxes and gave her the extra confidence she needed!

> **My dopamine was high, as it made me feel good helping someone who was struggling with their hair, especially when I was struggling with my own hair.**

However, when it came to recommending products for her, I was baffled with what to do. Do I give her one for thinning, frizz or volume? The best I could do was mix them up.

Coincidentally (or a sign), I started getting more clients with hair that was falling out, frizzy, thinning, and oily – and they were also in the age bracket for menopause. I started to have more and more conversations with them about what was happening and what we were going through. Before long, I started to put it all together. What I had been going through with my own hair, what that first client Natalie had been experiencing, and what I had seen with other clients since was all related to menopause.

Even though I realised this was most likely the cause, there was still no clear direction to fix the issues. I got stuck on what to recommend clients and what to even use for myself. What do I give a client who is having more than two issues and which products do I offer them that will help? For instance if I gave a client a shampoo for oily hair, this wouldn't benefit their frizzy hair, but if I gave them a serum for the frizziness, it would weigh their hair down. And none of these options would help their hair from falling out or becoming thinner. I started thinking, *this is ridiculous. How do I help someone who is coming to me but having more than one issue affecting them?* The more I tried with different products, the more apparent it became that I could only fix one problem but not the other.

One evening after work, I had a brainwave. I said to Pip, "There's nothing on the market for menopause-related hair changes. There needs to be a product or treatment for this." He was super supportive. He was like, "I think you are right, you could be onto something here."

Following Through

I had been hairdressing for 30 years and wanted to reward all my hard work with something big, but before this, I just couldn't work out what that big thing was. All I knew was that I wanted to give more and help people, as that is what I love to do. When the idea for the brand came through, I felt powerful, much like the strength I gained from prioritising myself. My mind felt equally strong, and anything seemed possible. It was like completing a jigsaw puzzle. This was a time for me to remember my true self and what I've always wanted to do. It provided instant direction.

> **I wanted to create this haircare brand to show both myself and other women that as we enter the menopausal phase, we don't need to give up on ourselves – whether it's our beauty, personality or power.**

When menopause causes changes in our hair, skin and body, it can bring a further sense of grief for who we used to be and a loss of confidence. The hair, skin and bodies that used to feel amazing now feel foreign, with an extra few hairs on our chins, sagging skin or a change of dress size.

The most challenging aspect is the societal expectation to look a certain way for our age. I don't see myself as an 'old' 50-year-old, nor do I relate to how my mother's generation perceived 50, but it seems there is still a strong societal pressure to maintain a youthful appearance. What hits the most through all of this change is the emotional impact of not feeling like *you*.

A loss of connection to one's self. If our hair or skin or what we are wearing doesn't feel right, then that's when self-worth begins to spiral because you don't like what you see. It really hit home when my client told me, "I just want my hair to feel like me again," and she's definitely not the only one. It's not just about beauty; it's a personal reconnection within ourselves.

This is what motivated me to start my brand, as there are women out there who need guidance and something that will give them the courage to move through this phase of their lives with confidence. It's also about honouring the journey, embracing the transformation that comes with it, and most importantly, knowing that you are not alone and you were never meant to disappear. I want women to feel a sense of ownership when they reach for it. It's a reminder that every woman matters and at this stage of life, they are still powerful and their identity hasn't faded but actually has gotten stronger.

This was something that I wanted to do for other women, but also for myself.

I wanted to show my family that I am a fighter and inspire my children that anything is possible and for them to be proud of me. I also wanted to create a message for the younger generation as well, including my three daughters and my son, that extra support is necessary to have when it comes to their turn or supporting their partners through theirs. I want the next generation to enter this phase of life with tools, education and a community. We need to embrace menopause in all its messy glory and show our own girls that they need to embrace it even better than what we did – instead of fighting it and being angry with it all.

With all this in mind, I attended my social media content class the next morning and I reached out to the content creator who ran the class after and told her what I was thinking. Without saying too much, she sent me a link to a person she had heard of that could help me. When I came home from my class, I sent an email to set up a call. It all happened so fast. I jumped on the call the following day, pitching my thoughts but all the while thinking it was a stupid idea – *what the hell was I thinking?* Our 15-minute call turned into an hour-long meeting, as we were both gobsmacked to be speaking to another hairdresser who had been in the business for so long yet hadn't thought about this. I thought to myself that if I'm struggling to help clients with the years of experience I've had with hair, how can young apprentices be guided to offer the same support to their clients? There needs to be some sort of education about it all. There was a huge market for this, and I had an energy and excitement about it that I hadn't felt in years.

I often hear, "You're writing a book, building a brand, raising four kids and running a business, all while going through menopause? Isn't that a lot?" Yeah it can be a lot, and some days the fatigue is real. Menopause has taught me how precious my energy is and I have had to learn when to push, when to pause, and how to store up any energy I can. I don't have energy to waste on things that don't align with me anymore.

But something shifted…

When the idea for the brand and book came through, I felt powerful and like anything was possible. I embraced it, as I was healing and this was my destined journey. It was a time for me to remember who I really am and what I have always wanted to do. It provided me with instant direction.

I do still get tired, and when I haven't slept, I can get frustrated and my mind fills with noise – the mental chatter that accompanies hormones, responsibilities, emotions and life. I also had a lot of doubts about the brand, but I learned how to turn the fear into fuel. Instead of letting it all overwhelm me, I channelled it into research, writing and creating. If my mind was going to be busy, it may as well be building something meaningful. It became my escape, my release and my way of transforming chaos into clarity.

And the wildest part? As a kid I always dreamed of writing a book and being a hairdresser. I was obsessed with art, with creating and expressing something real. I didn't know how it would come together but now, through menopause of all things, it's happening.

It's like this whole chaotic hormonal transformation chapter was actually what forged me into the version of myself that could do what I was always meant to do.

Wait... I'm in Post-Menopause?

The other day, someone casually asked me, "So, when did you transition into post-menopause?"

I paused, blinked and thought... *Umm, good question.* For some reason, I always thought *post-menopause* was something that happened much later in life. I assumed it was just a label slapped on once you hit your 60s or beyond. *How brain-fogged and naive was I?* I hadn't realised that transitioning into post was when you don't have a period for longer than a year.

One of the biggest challenges during this whole thing wasn't actually the symptoms – it was the lack of education. My own, but also my husband's, my children's, and literally everyone else around me. How is it that we know how atoms work and not the female body?! (If you want to truly feel enraged about why exactly this is, research when they started allowing women to be part of clinical studies...). So after this conversation, I was curious (and slightly embarrassed), so I went down the research rabbit hole. What I found was both enlightening and confusing.

The three stages of menopause:

1. **Perimenopause:** This stage can begin anywhere from 8–10 years before menopause, usually when a woman is in her 40s. It can last for months or years. Symptoms vary from person to person, but generally include irregular periods, hot flashes, mood swings and trouble sleeping.

2. **Menopause:** Rather than a stage per se, menopause is a marked point when you haven't had a period for 12 months. The body has stopped releasing eggs and the level of estrogen produced has decreased.
3. **Post-Menopause:** This is the stage right after the 12 months and it lasts for the rest of the person's life. Symptoms may ease, but it varies between individuals and some symptoms could persist for several years after menopause.

So technically, I am in post-menopause. The word *post* makes it sound like it's over. Like we've crossed the finish line and now it's all smooth sailing from here. We're told that things 'should' get easier. That we'll feel *relief*. But what now? What actually happens when you've officially crossed the 'no more period' line? Do you get a badge of honour? A welcome pack? A little whisper in your ear saying, "Congratulations, you're all good now. Return to being yourself." No. What you get is silence. Fog. Some relief, maybe. Some days that feel more manageable. But more often, it's a mix of old symptoms reshaped, new ones you weren't prepared for, and a sense that you're now living in a body that doesn't always feel like home. Some symptoms shift. Others intensify. And some may continue indefinitely without proper care.

Things I wish I knew sooner about post-menopause:

1. **Symptoms don't always vanish:** They may change, yes, but many linger. If something feels off, it's not "just in your head." It's your body calling for attention.
2. **Support matters:** Whether it's your family, HRT, supplements, acupuncture, therapy, or simply having the right doctor, it matters to feel seen and heard.
3. **Identity shifts are real:** Post-menopause can feel like a loss, especially when youth and womanhood have been tied to periods and fertility. Give yourself time to grieve what was and make space for what is.
4. **You're not alone:** Millions of women are going through this right now. We're just not talking about it enough, so start the conversation!
5. **It's not too late:** To start a new chapter. To change your lifestyle. To reconnect with your body. To feel beautiful, strong, desirable, powerful. It's not too late to be whatever and whoever you want.

***

Not long ago, we had a family dinner followed by a movie night. Naturally it fell on me to do the bookings, the kind of invisible responsibility mothers carry without question. But after a day in the salon and talking all day, the brain can get a bit sluggish.. But it means a lot when the kids want family time, so I organised last-minute tickets and booked a place for dinner. When we arrived at our local cinema, I stepped confidently to the counter and gave my surname, even spelling it out. The lady looked puzzled and replied, "I can't find it."

I knew I had booked it, so I pulled out my phone for proof. And then my son read the tickets over my shoulder and said, "Mum, you booked the wrong cinema."

I froze. The tickets weren't cheap as we went Gold Class, and he was right – I had booked the wrong place. We had to repurchase the tickets, and while the lady kindly explained how I could get a refund, my family's response was a simple, "Mum, it's okay." They all were quiet for a change.

But inside, I felt so small. I felt stupid and embarrassed. I don't make mistakes. I'm the one who organises, who remembers, who holds the details together. It was more than a booking error, it was a crack in who I believed myself to be now. And that's exactly what menopause can feel like. I have always been the one to lead, and my son even calls me the CEO of the family. I am the reliable one, and then menopause comes along and I'm all of a sudden forgetful, lose track of my thoughts, or make small fuck ups that feel monumental.

The truth is that mistakes don't erase our worth. My family didn't love me less for booking the wrong cinema – they reassured me it was okay. So I've had to work on unlearning the pressure to be perfect and instead accept myself as human. Since then, it's about letting go of control. For example, on a family holiday, I used to hold all the passports and boarding passes and even fill out everyone's forms on the plane. Now, I trust everyone with their own and everyone does their own forms. Everyone also now orders their own meals at restaurants, and I've set boundaries with my mental load in general, including what questions I'll answer. Every mum knows what this is like – we're the home Google. Now when someone asks me a question that they can find out themselves, I say, "Sorry, I'm not Google, please find it yourself." It's all these little things that people might think are stupid, but it's about offloading to give my brain space to breathe.

For me, post-menopause feels like I'm wearing someone else's skin and still trying to figure out how to make it feel like my own again. Some days, I feel empowered. Other days, I feel ancient and make silly mistakes like the cinema.

> But through it all, I remember that I'm in control now.

If there's one silver lining to menopause, it's this: **No. More. Periods.**

That was hands-down the best part. No more tracking cycles on a calendar. No more counting days to avoid falling pregnant – or trying to make it happen. No more waking up doubled over with cramps. I got my period at the age of 10 and it all stopped at 45 – that's more than three decades of bleeding, bloating and backaches. If that's not enough service to womanhood, I don't know what is.

So yes, I celebrated. Quietly. Loudly. Internally. Externally. Whatever way I could. Despite the other challenges I now faced, it was freedom. But don't get me wrong, there was still a sad part of me that felt like my duty of being a woman was done and what my body was made to do had ended, which is why finding a purpose outside of it all was essential.

PART 3

Walking Through the Fire as a Warrior

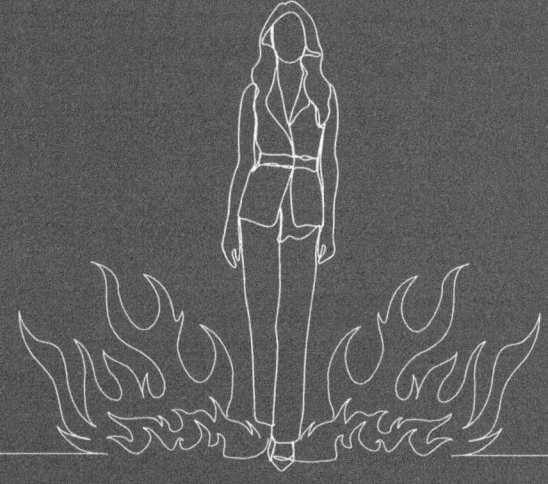

This is not the end of youth, it's the beginning of knowing yourself deeply.

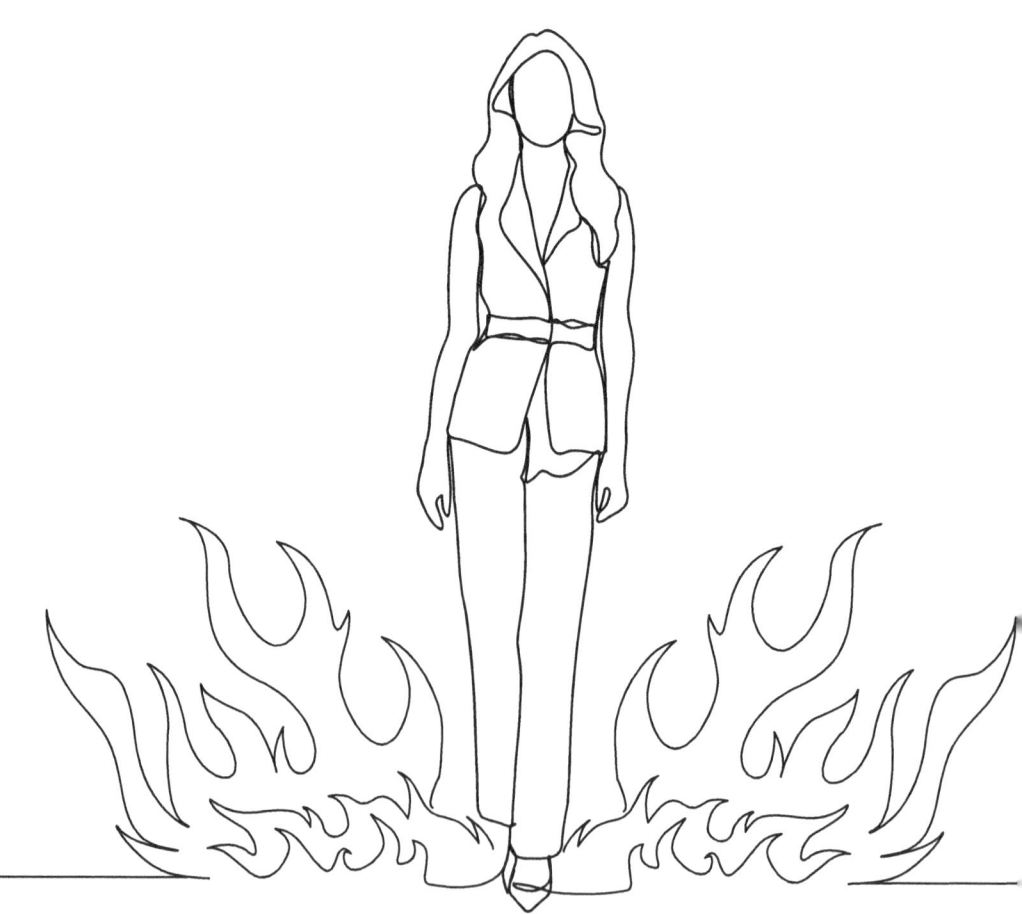

Menopause doesn't have to just be 'endured', it can be navigated and improved with a range of holistic wellness strategies, coping techniques and treatments. By taking back control over your life, you can truly thrive, rediscover joy, connect with yourself, and develop a profound sense of self throughout menopause. It's about trying to rebuild yourself again – putting the pieces back together, not just physically, but emotionally and mentally too. Think of the below chapters as your guide to reclaiming your power, finding clarity and embracing the undeniable woman you are becoming. We'll explore how each approach can alleviate symptoms, elevate your selfcare routine, and make you feel like yourself again (if not better!).

Haircare

When clients came in and were telling me they were losing hair, it wasn't just more strands falling out when brushing. I'm talking clumps of hair as I would comb it out, but then other clients would have short little bits of hair on the top where the hair strand had snapped. This didn't matter whether they had bleach in their hair or just a gloss colour. I also saw clients who believed they had come out of menopause but were still seeing that their hair was not the same as before they began – mainly when it came to texture. Clients who had really curly hair still had the curls, but they were a lot finer and each hair follicle was a lot softer – like cotton wool texture.

This isn't the only phase in our lives when our hair changes. When I got my period, my hair went from pretty straight to a ringlet mop of hair. I was completely lost on how to look after it, as my mum's hair was dead straight so she didn't know either. My kids laugh at my year 7 photo, as it was so frizzy, it's like I had a bird's nest on my head. I later taught myself to comb my hair in the shower and put a treatment in to tame the frizz, and I had really tight curls from then on until I gave birth to my first child. A few days after delivery, I washed my hair, styled it as normal, and of course, it started to fall out almost immediately. But that was expected – the real shock came when I woke up the next day to flat hair. Overnight, my hair had lost the tight curls and they had become a lot more loose and less defined. So menopause was the third time my hair had changed, and it was when I'd had enough of my hormones dictating how much I was able to feel like myself. Since I am a hairdresser, my hair felt like the most important thing to fix to get this feeling of 'myself' back, and it seemed like the easiest thing to be in control of.

Wendy the Brand

Wendy the Brand is truly more than just a line of hair products; it's a community, a warm conversation, and a heartfelt promise. A promise that you are seen, you are heard, and you are truly unstoppable. I poured my whole heart, and yes, a lot of late nights, into creating something really special just for us. Because, let's be honest, it felt like no one was really talking about what we go through or creating luxury haircare that targets exactly what menopausal women need. This brand comes from a place of genuine care and a deep desire to see every woman feel joyful, understood and confident.

Why does our hair seem to have a mind of its own during menopause? It really boils down to those shifting hormones. You might start noticing things like:

- **More breakage:** Your hair might feel a bit more delicate, snapping more easily than before.
- **Some thinning:** Your ponytail might feel a little less full or you see more strands than usual in your brush, on your clothes or falling out in the shower.
- **Unexpected frizz:** Suddenly, you brush your hair and it becomes a ball of frizz. No amount of hair product can get those strands smooth and flyaway free.
- **Feeling dry:** Your hair, which used to feel so soft, might now feel parched and brittle.
- **Scalp surprises:** An itchy, flaky, or even overly oily scalp can sometimes pop up as a new, uninvited guest.

These are all super common experiences and they're directly linked to our bodies adjusting to the new hormones. But just because they're common doesn't mean we have to just accept them! I knew there was an opportunity here to create products that targeted all these issues so that we didn't have 15 different bottles cluttering our shelves trying to get our old hair back.

Empowering women to get the look at home

One of the most powerful ways to serve women is to teach them how to use those products to transform their daily routines. Education is the missing link that turns hair and beauty care into a truly empowering experience. For too long, women have felt that salon-quality results are out of reach unless they book an appointment. But with the right guidance, tools and a step-by-step approach, women can learn to achieve confidence-boosting looks in the comfort of their own homes. This is where the educational side of Wendy the Brand comes in – bridging the gap between salon luxury and everyday accessibility.

Products alone can only go so far. Without the knowledge of how to use them effectively, women are often left frustrated, wasting time and money. Education transforms products from something they own into something they master. By sharing tutorials, techniques and professional insider tips, women begin to feel in control of their own beauty journey.

Wendy the Brand isn't just about amazing hair products, it's about being able to feel like the best version of yourself in a time when everything seems out of your control.

Community Support

While embracing the powerful transformation of menopause, it's so easy to feel isolated, like you're the only one experiencing these shifts. But I found immense solace and strength in sharing my journey – transforming my salon chair into a safe haven where women could connect, share and realise they weren't alone. We began to laugh together about how our husbands annoyed us, or something about the kids, and then it was like how we felt, whether it was good or bad.

> **The best medicine was laughing about it.**

We took the piss out of ourselves – our forgetfulness or what was annoying the shit out of us. This is when I really leaned into being able to relate to my friends to get through it, especially with one of my good friends in particular. She was always ahead of me by a year when it came to our babies and what we were going through with our kids, so she would go through it first and I would follow shortly later. As menopause got worse, thank God the social media content became funnier and more relatable. We would find memes and send them to each other. I would be sitting on the couch and burst out laughing with how much I could relate to the reel she had sent me and see how other people were also handling the tsunami that is menopause. From the reels detailing the extent of the outbursts to the ones describing our teens' phases of entitlement, they turned things that had really hurt me into something I could laugh at. Everything becomes less overwhelming when we do it together.

This is where my journey turned into more of an investigation into what could help me through the process. The community around me helped take the edge off when feeling a certain way or how my body is reacting to menopause, but it also made me realise that if everyone was feeling like this, there had to be ways to help. It became like an experiment of what worked for me and what didn't. It was like try it, see how you go, and if it worked, keep with it – if it doesn't, get back to researching and see what else can help.

More on Community from Kristy Borbas at Sacred Sisterhood Rising

My menopausal journey has been the hardest, most uneven road I've ever walked. The sleepless nights, the weight that wouldn't budge, the bone-deep aches, the mental fog, the anger and depression – all uninvited guests in my body's home.

Yet through this storm, I discovered something extraordinary: a portal to freedom.

Freedom from caring what others think. Freedom to ask, *Who am I hiding from? Is this really me? Is this all I've got left?* With potentially fewer years ahead than behind, I began questioning how I want to show up – as a mother, wife, sister, daughter and

WOMAN. What's truly shocking is the silence. Behind closed doors, we suffer through symptoms as if they're shameful secrets. When I sought help, I found a medical system that sees women up until they're 45 and then forgets us until 70 — as if the decades between hold no significance or medical relevance. We become second-class citizens, valued only during childbearing years, then discarded.

This realisation sparked my purpose: creating a community for women over 45. A space where nothing is taboo and where we can share what works, from natural remedies to HRT (which transformed my life), and what may not suit our needs. So I created Sacred Sisterhood Rising, which is a community that will love and accept you for exactly who you are and where authenticity is celebrated, spirituality is embraced, and transformation happens at the deepest level. This is a sanctuary for women ready to step into their next-level selves. Here, we weave together multiple wisdom traditions: astrology readings that illuminate your path, tarot that unlocks hidden insights, channelled messages from beyond the veil, and the rich tapestry of ancient feminine wisdom our ancestors practiced before these gifts were diminished and dismissed.

Sacred Sisterhood Rising is becoming a global community where the spiritual and practical blend seamlessly. We focus on embodiment work, including being fully present in your body, feeling all emotions without judgement, and releasing the traumas, patterns and ancestral burdens that have held us captive. This deep energetic healing creates space for your authentic self to emerge. Through our rituals, feminine empowerment practices, and sisterhood support, you'll learn to honour your intuitive guidance, claim your power and live life on your terms. This is a 6-month minimum journey, though most women who begin working with me never leave – they experience such profound transformation that they choose to stay.

I love guiding women back to themselves, helping them reconnect with their innate wisdom and learn to trust their inner voice. In our safe container, you'll discover parts of yourself long forgotten or never fully expressed.

No matter what your community looks like, it's important to have one to lift you up and provide support on the days you feel the most disconnected from yourself. When we are surrounded by like-minded people in a safe space, magic happens and lives transform in the most beautiful ways.

My Meno Menu

While I took a strike against cooking, I learned pretty quickly that I feel much better and more in control when cooking wholesome and nutritious meals. I actually do love cooking – when it's not a chore – so I delved into creating dishes that were going to support me the best during this transition. When my body felt depleted, my mind would quickly follow suit, leading to that crushing fatigue, brain fog, and just feeling so much more emotionally sensitive. Focusing on nourishing my body with good food and plenty of water became crucial, especially when I was experiencing those fluctuating energy levels, hot flashes or just feeling utterly 'zombified' and disconnected. Your body will tell you what it needs – we just have to learn to listen.

There were weeks when I couldn't even face the kitchen. The thought of cooking felt like a chore that required a mental strength I simply didn't have. While my head was everywhere, the *extra thought* of figuring out what to make every night was a total drag. I didn't want another decision. Not one more thing on my already overloaded mental to-do list. I just wanted *someone else* to take over for once.

But slowly, something shifted.

I began to enjoy cooking again.

Not just doing it for the hell of it, but for the joy of creating. The passion returned. The connection to food as a form of expression, of comfort, of grounding – it all came back to me.

> **Glimpses of my real self started to show when I was doing what I enjoyed the most: cooking for people and sharing dishes with friends and family.**

Growing up, food was a way to get family together, just like a community, to share our stories and enjoy the food as well as the company. I started finding the latest restaurants and I would have to try. Japanese was definitely my fave and as long as there was gluten-free on the menu, I was happy. I would say to my husband, "I have found a new restaurant – shall we try?" It wasn't just about enjoying the food and reconnecting with each other, it became about how I could recreate these dishes and bring joy and excitement back to the kitchen. I would go home and put my own spin on it and recreate it.

I was recently on a photoshoot for my brand, and we had set up this dreamy, playful scene in a kitchen: women in their PJs enjoying the quiet ritual of cooking for themselves. I had prepped all the food the night before and I planned what I wanted to have in the scene – beautiful, nourishing, feel-good dishes that made the kitchen feel warm and alive.

My brand manager was there, casually observing – until I started prepping, cooking, arranging. And suddenly… he froze. He just stood there, staring at the food, taking in the smells, the energy, the flow of it all. And then he blurted out, "Wendy, what the fuck… this is *so* good." It was like he had never seen this side of me before. Like my cooking flipped a switch in his head. I think he was mind-blown by what I dished up. His brain went into overdrive. He started thinking of new ways to integrate this into my new brand. Bigger ideas. Bigger vision. Deeper connection to the brand we're building. Because he finally saw something I had almost forgotten about myself: I'm not just a hairdresser or a writer or a mum – I'm a creator. And food is just another way I tell stories. And the best thing is that it's real food – food we as hormonal women want to indulge in.

One of my favourite dishes to make now is my hormone-loving greens and maple salmon bites. It's gluten-free and high in protein, but it's also really beneficial for menopausal women because salmon provides Omega-3s, which reduces inflammation and supports mood and skin hydration. The broccolini and zucchini also aid in estrogen balance, the feta and almonds provide calcium and magnesium, and the lime and balsamic glaze provide bright flavours without adding excessive amounts of salt and sugar.

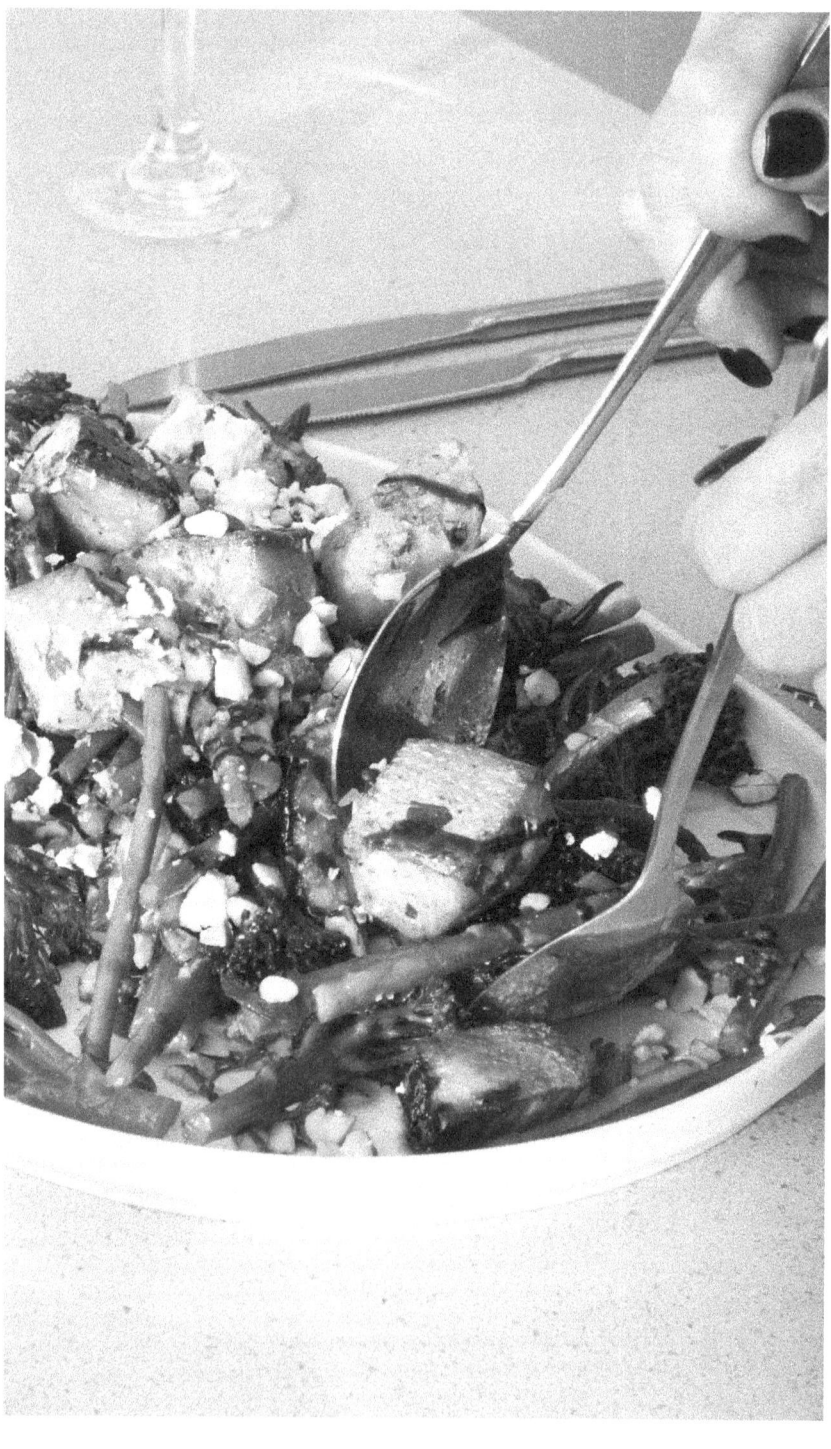

HORMONE-LOVING GREENS & MAPLE SALMON BITES

For the salmon:
2 salmon fillets, skin off and cut into bite-sized cubes
1 tbsp honey
1 tbsp maple syrup
Juice of 1 lime
A pinch of smoked paprika and garlic powder

For the greens:
1 bunch broccolini
1 small zucchini, sliced
1–2 tbsp olive oil
½ tsp red chilli flakes
Sea salt and cracked pepper
¼ cup crumbled feta
2 tbsp toasted flaked almonds
Balsamic glaze (to drizzle)

Marinate the salmon in honey, maple syrup, lime juice and seasoning for 15–20 mins.

Bake in a preheated oven at 180°C (fan forced) for 12–15 mins until golden and flaky.

Pan-fry the broccolini and zucchini in olive oil with chilli flakes, salt and pepper.

Arrange greens on a serving platter or bowl.

Top with crumbled feta, toasted almonds and a drizzle balsamic glaze.

Add salmon bites on top or serve separately in a bowl.

Holistic Coach

I started seeing Steve about 5 years ago when I was introduced to him by a client. He is very knowledgeable about the mind and body, and he is continually researching what is happening next to our bodies. When I walk in, he will study my stance and ask pointed questions before telling me what I need – nailing it every time.

When I saw Steve for the first time, he told me that he was aware I'd come for help with my weight and that he would help me if I wanted him to, but if I didn't want to do it for myself, then he couldn't help me. I remember getting in the car and crying, but it was the truth I needed at the time. That's how I lost weight in a healthy manner, steered by Steve, and this was before perimenopause began. Now he looks after my aches and pains, helps me when my immune system is low, guides me to the right podcasts for what I need at the time, and does acupuncture sessions with me. I like the fact that he is personal and only an email away, and when it comes to advice for me or the children, Steve always advises me on the best options and what to do. Having someone I can trust in this holistic way has been endlessly beneficial to my health and wellbeing throughout this journey, as they're like your personal life coach and aren't afraid to tell you what you need to hear to get shit done. Let's just say each appointment switches between physical or internal issues.

More from Steve at Effortless Superhuman

Menopause, a natural and inevitable phase in a woman's life, marks the end of her reproductive years. This transition is accompanied by a complex interplay of hormonal, physical and emotional changes that can significantly impact a woman's overall wellbeing. Understanding the multifaceted nature of menopause is crucial in developing a comprehensive approach to managing its effects.

At the core of the menopausal experience is the gradual decline in the production of estrogen and progesterone by the ovaries. This hormonal shift leads to a variety of symptoms, including hot flashes, night sweats, vaginal dryness, mood changes and sleep disturbances. While some women may sail through this transition with minimal disruption, others may face a more challenging journey, requiring a deeper understanding and proactive management of their symptoms.

Emerging research highlights the pivotal role of the gut microbiome in shaping the menopausal experience. The gut microbiome, the diverse community of microorganisms residing in the digestive system, plays a crucial role in various aspects of health, including estrogen metabolism, bone density, weight management and mood regulation. A balanced gut microbiome can help mitigate the severity of menopausal symptoms and support overall wellbeing during this life stage.

This can be achieved through a combination of dietary choices, probiotic supplementation and lifestyle modifications. A diverse, plant-based diet rich in fibre, fermented foods and nutrient-dense whole foods can help nurture a thriving gut ecosystem.

Complementing this dietary approach with regular physical activity, stress management techniques and mindful self-care can further support the gut-hormone axis and alleviate menopausal symptoms.

Beyond the gut-microbiome connection, other lifestyle factors can also significantly impact the menopausal experience. Factors such as metabolic disease, poor dietary choices, sedentary lifestyle and excessive alcohol consumption can exacerbate the symptoms of menopause, including hot flashes, mood swings and increased cardiovascular and metabolic risks. Adopting a holistic approach that addresses these lifestyle factors can empower women to navigate the menopausal transition with greater ease and resilience.

The team at ES uses a holistic, integrative approach to helping women who are pre-menopausal, menopausal or post-menopausal. This personalised approach includes understanding the current lifestyle factors that may be impacting the woman's overall health. Factors such as sleep, stress, daily activities, weekly exercise, current nutritional habits, medications, supplementation, personal care products, water quality and food quality. These 'basic' principles play a significant role in determining how easily a woman progresses through menopause.

In many cases, advanced testing is required to gain a deeper understanding of what may be driving a woman's menopausal symptoms. This may include advanced blood testing, DNA testing, gut microbiome testing, hormone tests and more. This detailed approach and individual care drives the success we have with our clients.

Ultimately, menopause is a multifaceted experience that requires a personalised and comprehensive approach. By understanding the intricate relationship between hormonal changes, gut health and lifestyle factors, women can work closely with their healthcare providers to develop a tailored plan that addresses their unique needs and supports their overall wellbeing during this transformative phase of life.

> **With a holistic perspective and proactive self-care, the menopausal journey can become an opportunity for growth, self-discovery and a new chapter in a woman's life.**

Pilates

For me, reformer Pilates was a quiet yet profound turning point. When I found myself in a hole, the simple act of moving my body became a lifeline. While it is simple in theory, we know that it can be one of the hardest things to do on a regular basis – but at the same time, I knew it would do wonders for my body. If you're feeling stiff, weak, lacking balance, or simply need to interrupt the noise in your mind, reformer Pilates can be an incredible reset. I found it allowed me to tune into my body, quiet my thoughts, and emerge with a blissfully clear head. I could feel each part of my body strengthening again, from my joints to my glutes, as well as my neck. It's particularly beneficial when you feel physically weak or disconnected from your own body, offering a gentle yet effective way to rebuild strength and centredness.

In saying this, I started at the beginners class and it got me *good*. I found it very challenging (and I was a bit embarrassed by how off-balance I was!). But I pushed through and now it is often the highlight of my day. So my advice for starting is to go in with no expectations, just a hope that it might help. Don't be embarrassed if you feel awkward or wobbly at first; everyone starts somewhere. Just keep going, one session at a time. Remember what it felt like to bounce out of that studio (even if you are sore), and you'll soon reap the benefits of your work.

By Afterglo Pilates

Reformer Pilates can be a great addition for women navigating the ups and downs of perimenopause and menopause. Pilates can help strengthen the body while providing much-needed support during this time of change. The reformer machine offers controlled resistance, which can be really beneficial for building strength and stability in the core, legs, and back. This is especially important as hormonal shifts can sometimes lead to decreased muscle mass and bone density.

On top of that, Pilates emphasises breathing and mindfulness, which can help manage the stress and anxiety that often accompanies these hormonal changes.

> **Women might find that focusing on their breath and movement not only strengthens their bodies but also calms their minds.**

Plus, the low-impact nature of reformer Pilates makes it accessible for those who might be dealing with joint pain or other discomforts. It's a fantastic way to reconnect with your body, boost your mood, and feel empowered during a time that can often feel overwhelming.

Strength Training

I haven't fully embraced strength training yet as I feel I'm not ready for it, but my goal is to continue doing Pilates and eventually build up to it. When you're feeling physically drained, weak, or simply not like yourself, the idea of intense exercise can feel completely overwhelming, so it's important to ease into it and do what feels right for you. But building strength is key to combating muscle loss, maintaining bone density, and boosting metabolism, all of which menopause can really mess with. It's a practice I'm looking forward to adding to my exercise routine, and one I know will make me regain a sense of physical power. And I know that when I'm ready, Clair and her team will be able to guide me into a program suited for me.

More from Clair Armstrong at PWR Fitness

Consider this period of your life an incredible change that is life growth. The opportunity to be strong in both mind and body. Learn to love STRENGTH – this will be your friend to support you both physically and mentally and to be powerful in all aspects of your life. Fuel and move your body to empower yourself. Consider this aging period as the time to embrace the best version of yourself.

Exercise, and in particular strength training, is one of the most important aspects of your overall health, especially during menopause. This is why it's integral to adopt an exercise regime that is specific to menopausal women, as it will help tackle the hormonal changes that can affect bone density, muscle mass, metabolism, and cardiovascular health. It's important to create a well-rounded exercise program that includes resistance, aerobic, flexibility and balance training to target common menopausal concerns like muscle decline, weight gain, bone density, mood swings and joint pain.

Remember, be kind to yourself and listen to your body! Menopausal fatigue and joint sensitivity vary and are different for everyone, so adjust intensity as needed. Hydrate well and consider calcium and vitamin D for bone support. Work with a qualified and knowledgeable trainer initially to learn proper form and avoid injury. Stay consistent – just 15–20 mins per day has long-term benefits.

Lastly and most importantly, talk to your friends and family. Support each other and wrap your arms around the women who know and love you the most and enjoy this 'life growth' journey together.

Kinesiology

I was trying everything to see what would work, and I still felt this emotional emptiness from the endless voices in my head and the brain fog. That's when I branched out to kinesiology, seeking a deeper cleanse. When I'm feeling heavy, drained, or as if old traumas and emotional blockages are holding me back, I find that kinesiology brings a sense of release and a feeling of lightness. It's a way to rebalance and shift any blocked energy.

One of my clients recommended me to Cherie, and I went in open-minded, as I had never done anything like this before. But going in with a sense of being open will give you a better experience instead of arriving with a negative vibe. I remember getting off the massage table and losing my balance because I felt so light, and I left feeling like my mind and body were emptied, and honestly, it was a bizarre yet amazing sensation.

I seek out my kinesiologist when I feel particularly triggered, overwhelmed by emotional turmoil, or simply when I'm ready to let go of old patterns. We hold a lot of ancestral trauma in us and Cherie is guiding me to remove this through sessions to help me move forward. Riding the wave in menopause has forced me to tune in more to my mind and body. I have to stop and think about what I need and how I can help myself. To start, I'd say approach it with an open mind, find a practitioner you trust, and be prepared to engage in a conversation about your life, your challenges, and what you hope to release. The affirmations and energetic work can be deeply transformative, leaving you feeling incredibly light and more balanced.

By Cherie Daniel BSc, BN, Advanced Diploma Kinesiology

Over the years, I've seen how kinesiology energy work can be a deeply supportive tool for women during menopause in helping with symptoms such as hot flashes, poor sleep, weight gain, anxiety, depression, emotional ups and downs, libido and intimacy issues, brain fog and fatigue – all of which can significantly affect our quality of life.

Kinesiology is a therapy that studies the muscles to identify unbalances. It is a gentle whole-body approach that helps bring your system back into balance – physically, emotionally and energetically. There are five major ways kinesiology can help women going through this important life shift.

Helps the body rebalance hormones naturally

The diminishing hormone production changes that occur during the stages of menopause affect the entire body. I use muscle testing to assess stress in the endocrine system, including the:

- Ovaries (even post-menopause, their energy can still affect you)
- Adrenals (they take over some hormone production after menopause)
- Thyroid and pituitary glands (which often struggle under stress)

By identifying where your body is out of balance, I can apply gentle corrections and activate acupressure points to help your hormones regulate more smoothly.

Releases stored emotions

Menopause isn't just a physical transition, it's emotional and spiritual too. Many women experience unexpected waves of grief, irritability, anxiety, depression, or even a sense of losing themselves.

In a kinesiology session, I often find that emotional patterns are stored in the body and may be linked to specific organs (like the liver holding anger or the kidneys holding fear). We work together to gently release these using:

- Emotional stress release (ESR)
- Meridian tapping and affirmations
- Vibration resonance with tuning forks
- Flower essences and energy techniques

This process can feel like a reset that helps you feel lighter, calmer, clearer and more like yourself again.

Soothes common menopausal symptoms

Hot flashes, night sweats, insomnia, low energy and fatigue can all be made worse by the imbalances in your meridians or stress on your nervous system.

One area I focus on is the triple heater meridian, which governs the stress and hormonal systems. When it's overactive, your body stays in 'survival mode' and symptoms can intensify. Balancing this, along with other key meridians like the heart, liver and kidney, often brings noticeable relief. It's not just about managing symptoms, it's about helping your energy flow freely again.

Calms the nervous system

So many women I see are running on empty, especially during perimenopause and beyond. The nervous system can become overstimulated, leading to anxiety, overthinking, poor sleep and overwhelm/burnout.

In my sessions, I use kinesiology tools to calm the sympathetic nervous system (fight/flight) and support the parasympathetic nervous system (your 'rest and restore' state). This leaves clients feeling lighter, calmer and more centred in their bodies.

Empowerment and self-care

Kinesiology also encourages women to tune into their body's wisdom to understand the root causes of symptoms, reclaim energy and vitality, and navigate the emotional and spiritual aspects of midlife transformation.

Energy work for menopause is a whole person approach — physical, emotional, energetic and spiritual. It doesn't treat menopause as a problem but rather supports women through a powerful life shift with insight, balance and empowerment.

As a side note, I personally have experienced the frustration of lack of healthcare system support, as well as the lack of knowledge of all the symptoms that women experience. For example, when I was in my early 40s, I had plantar fasciitis, was taking longer to recover after workouts, and felt frustrated with stiffness, soreness and fatigue post-workout. These were signs of estrogen loss. Urinary tract infections may also be related to estrogen loss, as well as changes in bacterial flora and pH in the vagina to prevent irritation and dryness. This has such a big impact on relationships and intimacy and is generally very poorly addressed. Much more information and support needs to be available to women to help them understand their bodies holistically and navigate this journey with ease, grace and joy.

Skin Treatments and Cosmetic Injections

As I navigated the changes that came with menopause, my skin certainly told a story of its own, reflecting those shifts in hormones and overall wellbeing. What hit home for me was how my face changed and looked old overnight. It was like everything felt extra elasticated and droopy, and a few more wrinkles had been added to my eyes and forehead. I felt like I couldn't even recognise myself in the mirror anymore. For me, investing in skin treatments and even cosmetic injections became a part of feeling more like myself again, addressing concerns like dryness, loss of elasticity or those unwelcome lines. I lost a lot of collagen, which sagged my skin at a rapid rate. Treatments can be a valuable tool when you feel your external appearance doesn't quite match the vibrant person you are inside, or when you simply want to feel more confident and refreshed. It's truly about personal choice and what makes you feel good.

A quick note: injectables aren't for everyone and this isn't a recommendation, but simply something I choose to do and something that makes me feel more confident within myself. I still wanted to look as natural as possible without the extra roadmaps on my forehead. It's important to do your research, consult with qualified professionals, and understand all aspects of the procedure. My advice here is to explore what makes you feel comfortable and confident in your own skin, always prioritising your health and wellbeing.

By Jemma Gleeson at Skin Societé

I'm Jemma Gleeson, a registered nurse, cosmetic injector, and the proud owner of Skin Societé in Karrinyup and Ellenbrook. I work closely with women of all ages, but I have a special interest in helping women experiencing the profound changes of menopause. For many of my clients, menopause feels like a loss of control over their skin, bodies and sense of identity. My mission is to help them understand what's happening beneath the surface and to offer expert care and aesthetic treatments that support both inner wellness and outer beauty.

At Skin Societé, we combine clinical precision, a detailed understanding of the anatomy, and your natural beauty to make you feel your very best. We specialise in advanced cosmetic injectables and skin treatments tailored to the unique physiology of midlife skin. But more importantly, we listen. We educate. We empower. Because menopause is more than a hormonal shift – it's a major life transition and we believe women deserve expert support through it all.

Hormones and skin health

The skin is a hormone-sensitive organ. Estrogen receptors are found in every layer, from the epidermis down to the dermis and fat layer. By understanding these changes, we can target treatments with precision.

Women in menopause often experience a wide range of skin and aesthetic changes, including:

- Thinning skin and loss of elasticity
- Wrinkles and fine lines
- Volume loss in the cheeks, lips and under eyes
- Dullness, dehydration and sensitivity
- Hyperpigmentation and melasma
- Acne or rosacea flare-ups
- Facial hair growth
- Redness and visible capillaries
- Sagging around the jawline and neck

These changes are more than cosmetic – they often affect a woman's confidence, relationships, and overall mental health.

Treatments tailored for menopausal skin

Anti-wrinkle injections

As estrogen drops, collagen production declines and the skin becomes thinner and more prone to creasing. Anti-wrinkle injections (neuromodulators like botulinum toxin) relax the muscles responsible for dynamic lines, such as crow's feet, forehead lines and frown lines. This not only smooths existing wrinkles but helps prevent deeper ones from forming.

Dermal fillers

With menopause comes the breakdown of collagen, elastin and facial fat. Hollowing around the eyes, sagging cheeks and thinning lips are common. Dermal fillers, typically made from hyaluronic acid, restore lost volume and reshape facial contours for a lifted, rejuvenated appearance.

Skin boosters

Think of skin boosters as injectable moisturisers. Rather than adding volume, they deeply hydrate the skin by delivering micro-injections of hyaluronic acid and other bioactive ingredients. This improves tone, elasticity and radiance without altering facial shape. You might have heard of Rejuran, which is one of the latest treatments available where salmon DNA (AKA sperm – weird, I know) is injected into the superficial layers of the skin to rebuild the tissue, making it smoother and stronger. As gross as it is, it's proving to be a revolutionary treatment in the market!

Biostimulators

Collagen-stimulating treatments and PDO threads don't just fill, they help your body rebuild itself. These biostimulators are injected into deeper layers of the skin, prompting gradual collagen regeneration over time. The results are subtle but transformative, continuing to give you better and better results over the course of 2 years.

Microneedling and radiofrequency (Fractional RF)

Fractional RF combines tiny needles with heat to stimulate tissue regeneration and firm lax skin. This dual-action treatment is ideal for menopausal skin that's losing elasticity and developing fine lines, sagging, or uneven texture.

Chemical peels

Our advanced medical-grade peels are tailored to your skin's needs – from light exfoliation to deeper pigment correction. It does so by encouraging cell turnover, which improves complexion over time and creates a healthy glow.

Menopause is often painted as a time of decline – but I see it differently. It's a time of self-rediscovery. A chance to reclaim your body, your beauty, and your sense of self on your own terms. Every woman deserves to look in the mirror and see someone she recognises and loves.

Lymphatic Draining Massage

I found immense relief in lymphatic drainage massages, especially when I was dealing with fluid retention, puffiness, inflammation and just a general need for relaxation. It's a gentle yet powerful technique that provides relief for stagnant energy in the body. This is a practice I turn to when my body feels heavy, sluggish or when I simply need a moment of calm and physical release. And I definitely noticed that my lymphatic system was extra sluggish while in perimenopause. The place I go to has a calming entry, a heated bed and headphones to listen to calming music. And that's all before the massage starts.

> It's pure bliss for my mind and my body.

By Vanessa from Lymphatic Massage Perth

Lymphatic drainage massage can be a valuable ally for women going through menopause, helping to ease common symptoms caused by hormonal fluctuations. As estrogen levels decline, many women experience water retention, swelling and bloating – especially in the legs, ankles and face. Lymphatic massage stimulates the flow of lymph, reducing fluid buildup and supporting the body's natural detoxification process. This technique can also help flush out excess hormones and metabolic waste, promoting better balance and overall health.

Beyond physical relief, lymphatic massage also supports emotional wellbeing. Menopause often brings stress, anxiety and sleep disturbances, and this massage activates the parasympathetic nervous system to induce deep relaxation. Women frequently report improved sleep, reduced irritability and a greater sense of calm after sessions. Additionally, the boost in circulation can improve skin tone and reduce puffiness, offering a rejuvenated and healthier appearance.

Sound Healing

Before I attended the sound healing retreat, I started going to sound healing classes, where I got to listen to the sound of the bowls, breathe deep, and go to a place to feel calm, relaxed and my brain got to rest. I entered with an open mind and was greeted with candles and a mattress to lie on that was as soft as a cloud. I found this so helpful for emptying my thoughts, so then I thought why not try a retreat? I finally committed to one at a time when I was feeling a deep emotional emptiness, despite physical improvements.

When feeling overwhelmed, emotionally numb, disconnected or simply craving peace and quiet to interrupt the internal noise, sound healing can be a powerful reset. It's a practice I turn to when my mind is racing, my emotions feel stuck or I'm yearning to feel something again, to reconnect with my inner self. You don't need to know exactly what you're looking for; sometimes, the experience itself reveals what you need.

> **I found it took me to a whole new place, helping my thoughts quieten and allowing me to tune into my body, leading to a blissfully clear head and an emotional shift.**

I also found it helpful to calm my nervous system, as I have never had anxiety before but peri brought on a slew of anxiety and a sense of unease. Sound healing provides rare relief from this.

This isn't for everyone, and some people can't switch off in just one session. It took me a few classes to be able to get in the zone and take me to my happy, calming place, so don't give up if you feel like it's not getting you what you need at the start. Definitely give it a good go and find a practitioner you can connect with.

By Sanchia from Soundhealingperth

This phase of life brings immense change – physically, emotionally, mentally and spiritually. For many women, it can be a disorienting time marked by symptoms like brain fog, a racing mind, sleep disruptions, hot flushes, mood swings and a deep sense of inner shifting. Sound healing offers a nurturing, non-invasive way to reconnect with the body, soothe the nervous system and come home to self.

How sound healing helps

1. **Nervous system regulation:** Sound frequencies slow down brainwaves, guiding the body out of 'fight or flight' and into 'rest and repair'. This helps reduce stress, overwhelm, and that feeling of being 'wired but tired'.
2. **Mental clarity and brain fog relief:** Gongs, crystal bowls and tuning forks produce harmonics that can quiet a racing mind and improve mental clarity. Many women report leaving a session feeling clearer, lighter and more grounded.
3. **Emotional balance:** Menopause can bring up old grief, identity shifts and mood swings. Sound healing creates a safe space for emotional release, supporting women to feel, process and let go.
4. **Sleep support:** The deep relaxation achieved in a session can significantly improve sleep quality – something many women struggle with during this time.
5. **Hormonal and energetic recalibration:** Though not a medical intervention, sound healing supports the endocrine system by

reducing cortisol levels, encouraging balance, and realigning the energy body (chakras), especially the sacral and heart centres – both of which are often activated during menopause.
6. **Spiritual connection and empowerment:** Menopause is often called 'The Second Spring' in Traditional Chinese Medicine. It's a powerful rite of passage. Sound healing helps women reconnect with their intuition, inner wisdom and power during this sacred transition.

How sound healing can relieve menopause symptoms

Sound healing sessions, often involving soothing instruments like Tibetan singing bowls, produce vibrations that can induce deep relaxation for participants. Emerging research indicates that these sound-based practices offer tangible benefits for women going through menopause. From easing stress and anxiety to improving sleep and mood, sound therapy provides a holistic, non-invasive way to support wellbeing during this transition.

Brain fog and cognitive clarity

Menopausal brain fog refers to memory lapses, difficulty concentrating and mental fatigue. Engaging in sound therapy (such as meditation with singing bowls or calming music) has been shown to encourage a state of mental clarity, stimulate neural connections and improve cognitive functions like attention and memory. In practice, women often report that focusing on soothing sounds quiets mental chatter and improves their concentration. Stress worsens brain fog, so the deep relaxation from sound therapy – which lowers stress hormones – can further sharpen the mind.

Stress reduction and nervous system regulation

Sound healing naturally helps dial down stress levels, as therapeutic sound triggers the body's relaxation response by activating the parasympathetic nervous system. This leads to measurable calming effects, including reduced stress hormone levels and lowered blood pressure and heart rate – objective signs of a soothed nervous system. Sound therapy's gentle vibrations essentially guide the body into 'rest-and-digest' mode, relieving physical tension and anxiety. By regulating the nervous system in this way, sound healing creates an inner environment of calm. Many women in menopause find that a simple 15-minute sound bath or listening session leaves them feeling centred and less reactive to stressors in daily life. Over time, this stress reduction can have a compounding positive effect on other symptoms and overall health.

Anxiety relief and calming racing thoughts

Stress, anxiety and racing thoughts often spike during menopause, manifesting as restless worry or an overactive mind (especially at night). Sound therapy is emerging as a gentle antidote to this anxiety. It works by establishing a deep state of relaxation and synchronising brain activity to calming sound. As soothing tones wash over the listener, the nervous system calms and racing thoughts begin to slow. Many practitioners observe that sound baths can quickly shift women from a state of overwhelm to one of peace and present-moment awareness. By focusing the mind on gentle tones, sound therapy draws attention away from past or future worries and into a tranquil 'here and now'. This not only alleviates anxiety in the moment, but can train the mind to find calm more easily over time. For menopausal women dealing with bouts of panic or looping thoughts, incorporating sound healing into their routine offers a simple way to cultivate mental calmness and emotional resilience.

Hormonal imbalance and recalibration

Sound healing may aid hormonal recalibration in several ways. First, it lowers cortisol, which is known to disrupt the endocrine system when persistently elevated, so keeping this stress hormone in check is crucial. This stress relief gives the body a chance to restore its hormonal equilibrium. Moreover, research and traditional practices suggest that certain sound frequencies might gently stimulate the glands (pituitary, adrenal, thyroid) that regulate hormone production. While more studies are needed, it's thought that vibrational sound can 'massage' these endocrine organs and encourage optimal function. Another key factor is sleep – quality sleep is vital for hormone regulation (e.g., nightly release of melatonin and growth hormone), and sound therapy often improves sleep (as discussed below), thereby supporting hormonal balance. Anecdotally, many women find the gentle vibrations of sound baths help 'reset' their internal rhythms.

Emotional regulation and mood support

Sound healing offers a nurturing tool for emotional regulation, helping stabilise mood in both scientific studies and real-world practice. Notably, a 2022 randomised controlled trial found that simply listening to music significantly reduced depression levels in postmenopausal women compared to controls.[1] Over 6 weeks, the women who had regular 15-minute music sessions reported lower overall menopause symptom scores and less depressive mood than those who didn't. This suggests that music (a form of sound therapy) can act as a natural antidepressant and mood booster. From a biochemical perspective, calming sound triggers the release of 'feel-good' neurochemicals – dopamine, serotonin, endorphins, even oxytocin – which promote relaxation and positive feelings. Concurrently, sound therapy reduces stress hormones like cortisol, which are linked to irritability and mood swings. Together, these shifts create a more stable emotional state.

Improved sleep quality

Sound healing can be remarkably effective in promoting restful sleep during this transition. The gentle, repetitive sounds used in practices like sound baths, meditative music or white noise can lull the brain into a relaxed state conducive to sleep. The calming effect of sound is central to these benefits: music therapy has a long history of promoting relaxation and triggering endorphin release, which helps reduce the anxiety, pain and stress that often interfere with sleep. Sound healing likely aids sleep architecture as well by promoting slower breathing and a drop in heart rate as one listens, mimicking the natural physiological changes of falling asleep. And better sleep leads to better hormone regulation, sharper cognition and steadier moods the next day. Therefore, integrating calming sound rituals at night (like soft music, nature sounds or singing bowl recordings) can be a simple yet effective strategy to combat menopausal insomnia and restore rejuvenating rest.

Additional Holistic Techniques to Support Your Journey

The above are the holistic techniques that I have personally used and found to be beneficial, but other options include yoga, talk therapy, reiki, acupuncture, meditation, art, swimming, running, and anything else you can think of! No matter what you choose, the key is to tap into your creativity, restore your body's strength, and calm the mind.

Mind-Body Practices
Meditation
It's not about emptying your mind but rather observing it without judgement. Think of it as a mini-vacation for your brain! Practices like mindfulness, guided imagery, and simple relaxation techniques can be incredibly powerful for reducing stress and helping you focus on the present moment.

Yoga
More than just stretching, yoga is a fantastic way to reconnect with your body, build strength and find a sense of calm.

Tai Chi and Qigong
These ancient Chinese practices focus on slow, deliberate movements and breathing that help cultivate a serene energy within. It's a gentle way to move your body and quiet your mind.

Breathwork
Never underestimate the power of your breath! Consciously controlling and regulating your breathing can be a surprisingly effective tool for managing stress, calming anxiety and even boosting your energy.

Physical Therapies
Acupuncture
This ancient practice involves placing very thin needles into

specific points on your body. It might sound a bit prickly, but many women find it incredibly effective for relieving pain and easing various menopausal symptoms. It's all about balancing your body's energy pathways.

Massage therapy

A good massage is a powerful tool for promoting relaxation, reducing muscle tension and improving circulation. A little kneading can go a long way in soothing both body and soul.

Chiropractic and osteopathic manipulation

These manual therapies focus on your musculoskeletal system, particularly your spine. They can help ensure everything is aligned and moving as it should, which can be a real game-changer for aches and stiffness.

Energy and Arts Therapies
Reiki

This Japanese technique is all about channelling universal life energy through touch to promote stress reduction and healing. It's a gentle way to restore balance and harmony within your system.

Art therapy

Picking up a paintbrush, molding some clay, or simply colouring in can be incredibly therapeutic. Art therapy uses the creative process of art-making to improve your physical, mental and emotional wellbeing. It's about the process, not the end result.

Music therapy

Whether you're listening, singing or even trying your hand at an instrument, music therapy encourages expression through sound and can be a powerful tool for emotional release and connection.

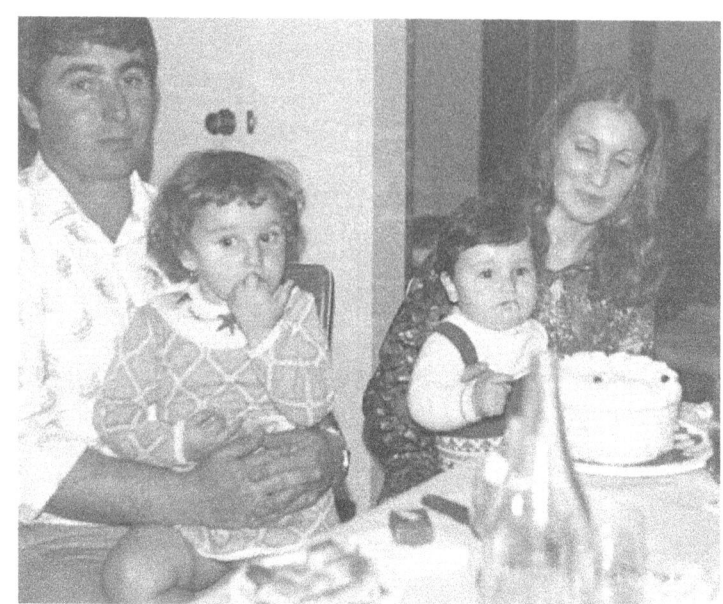
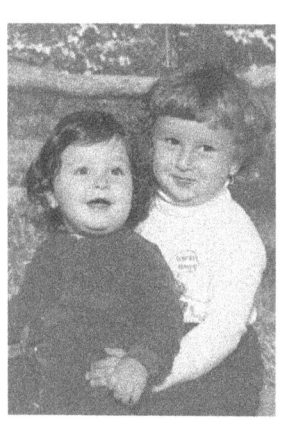
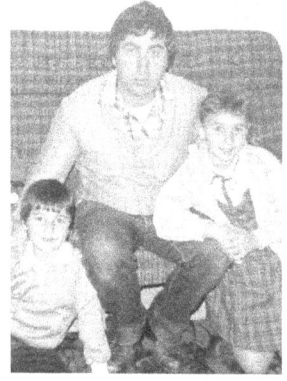
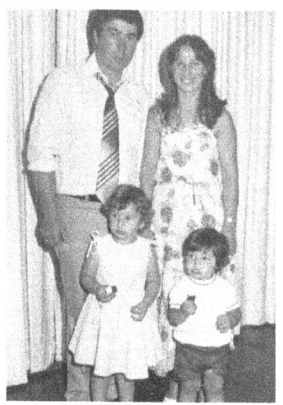
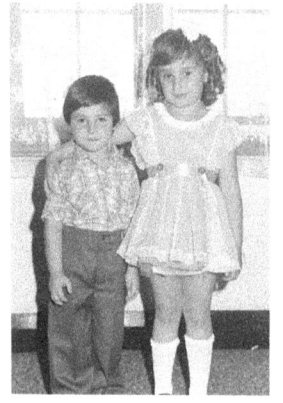
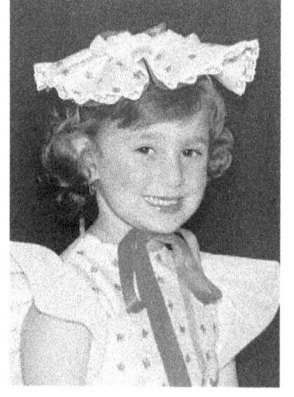
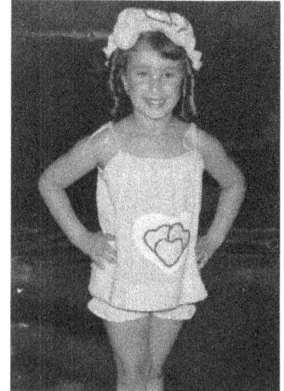

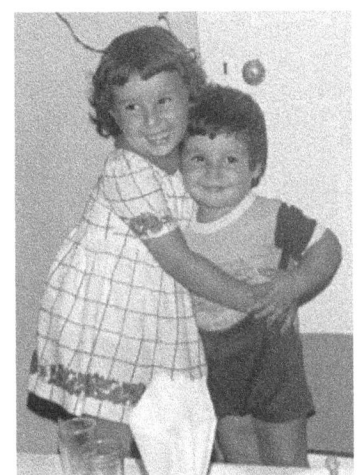
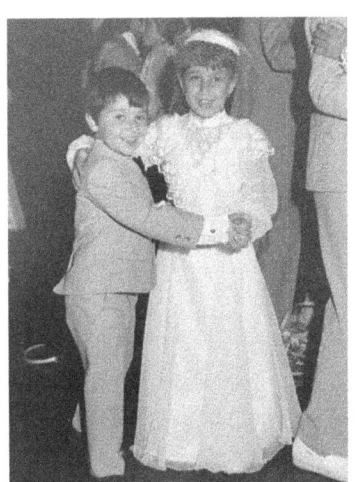
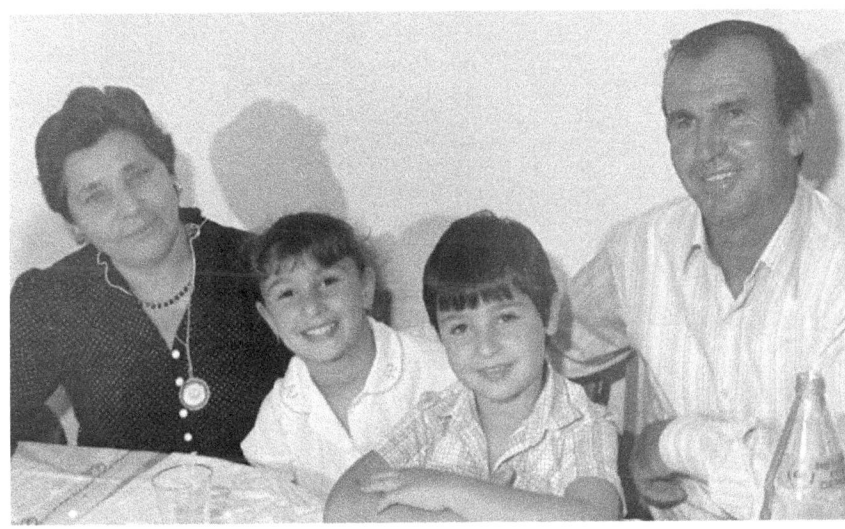
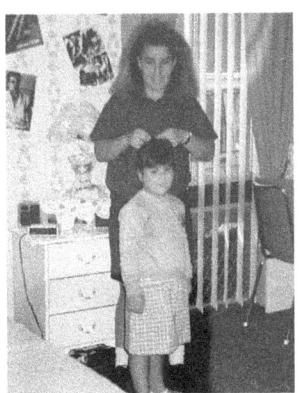
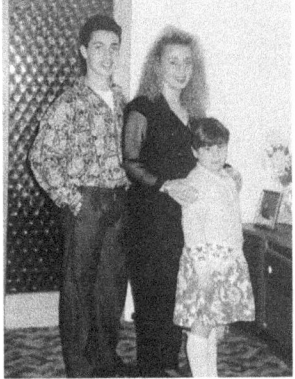
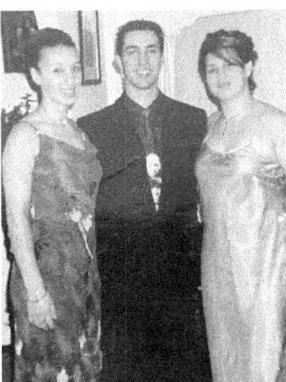

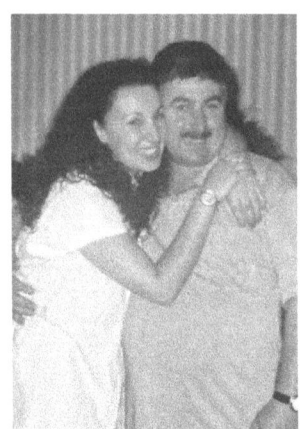
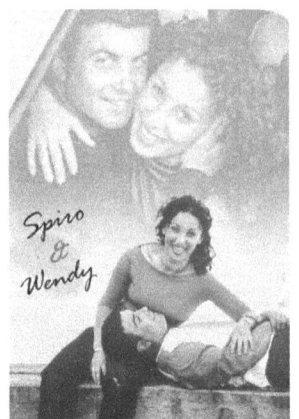
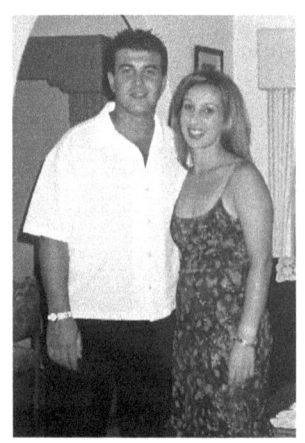
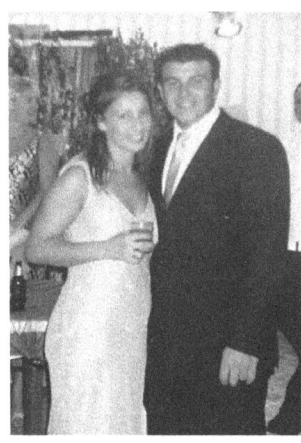
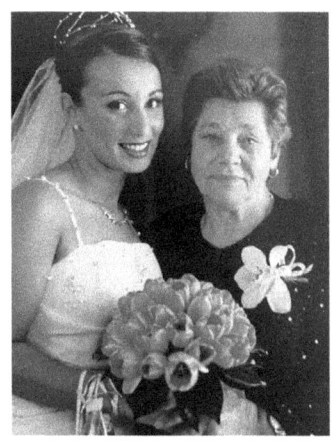
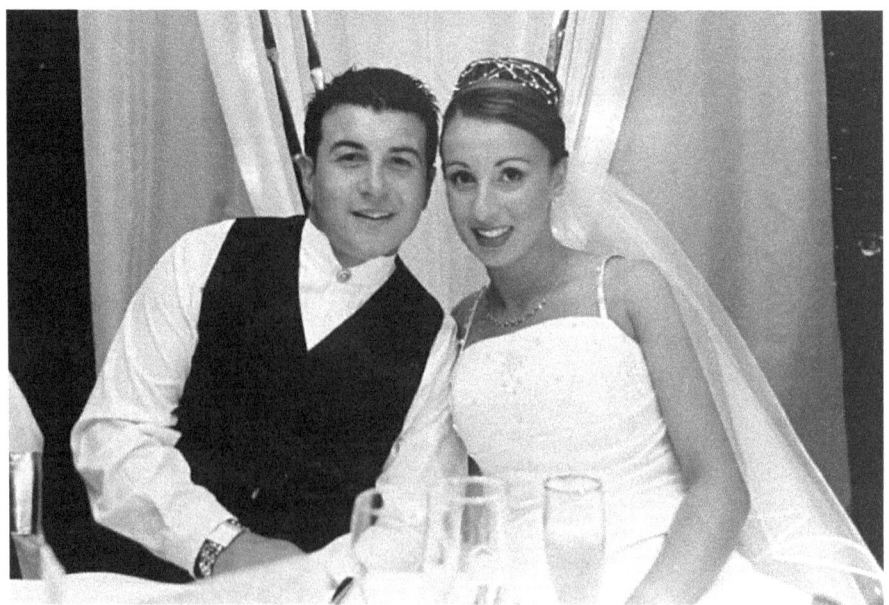

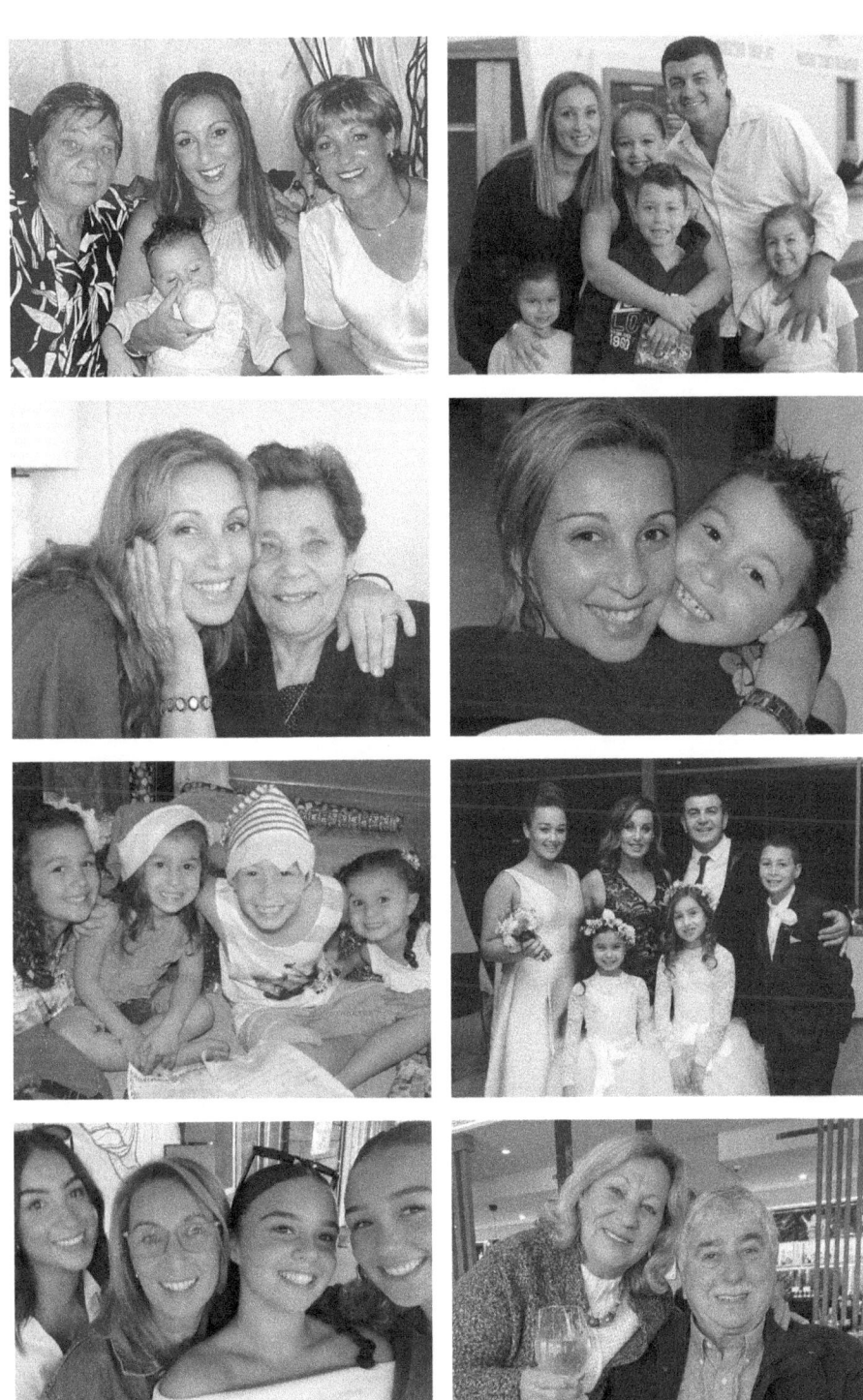

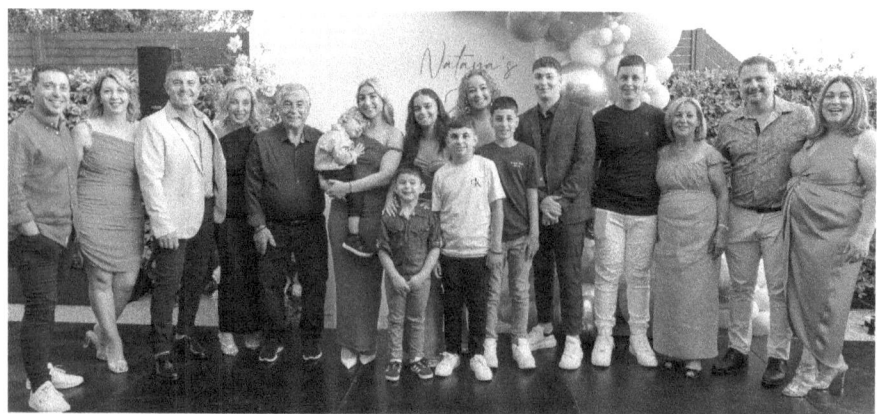
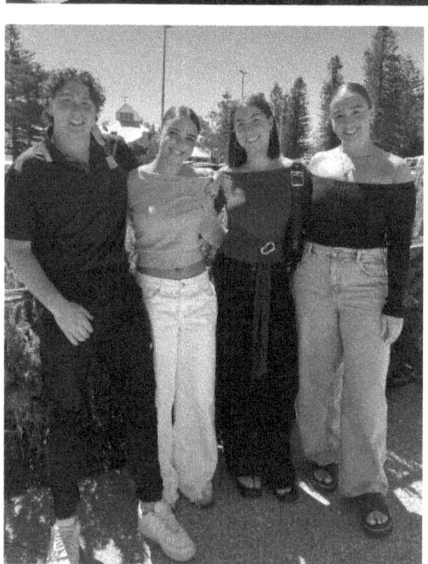
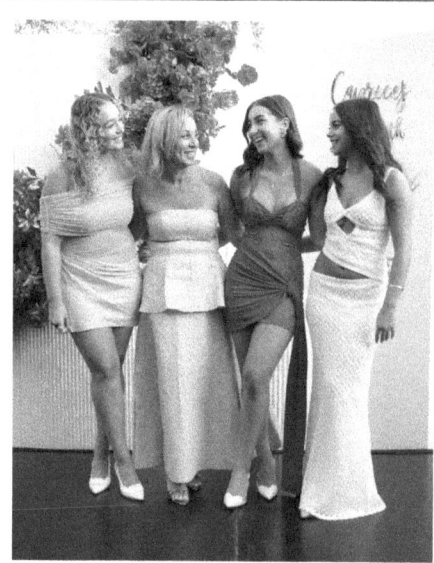
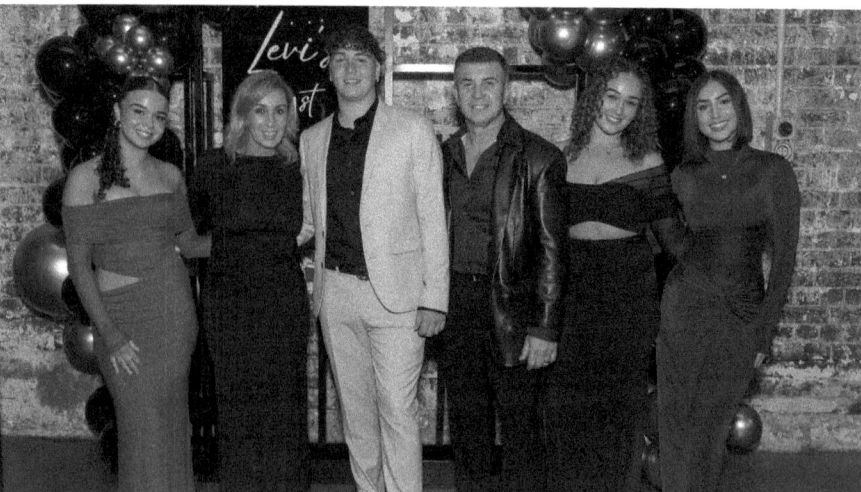

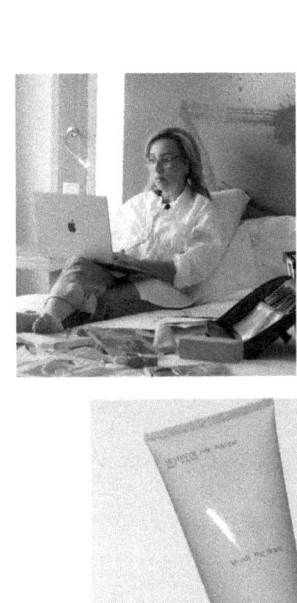
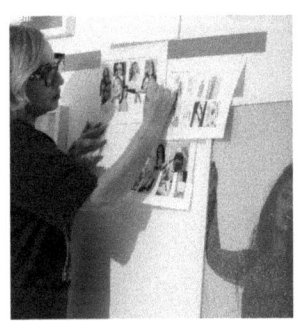
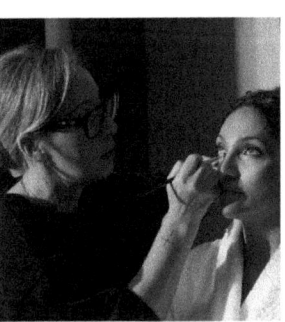
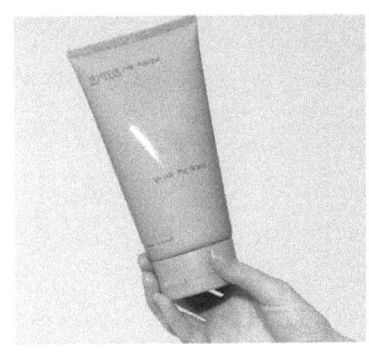
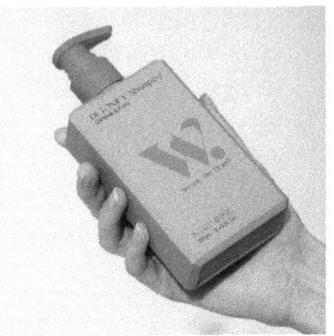
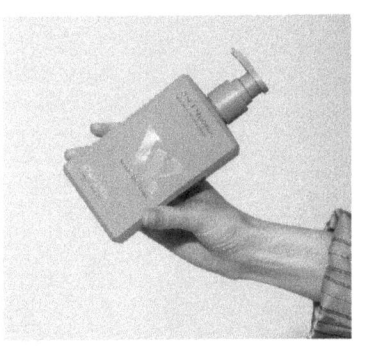
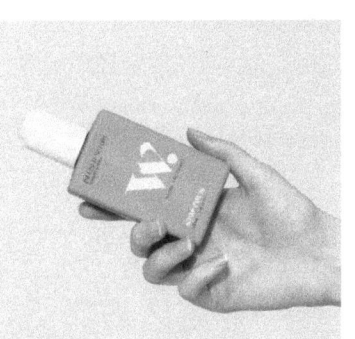
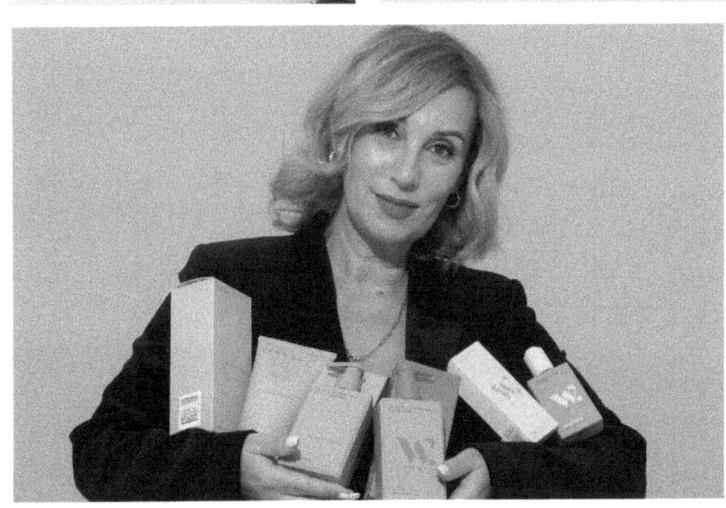

PART 4

Navigating Relationships

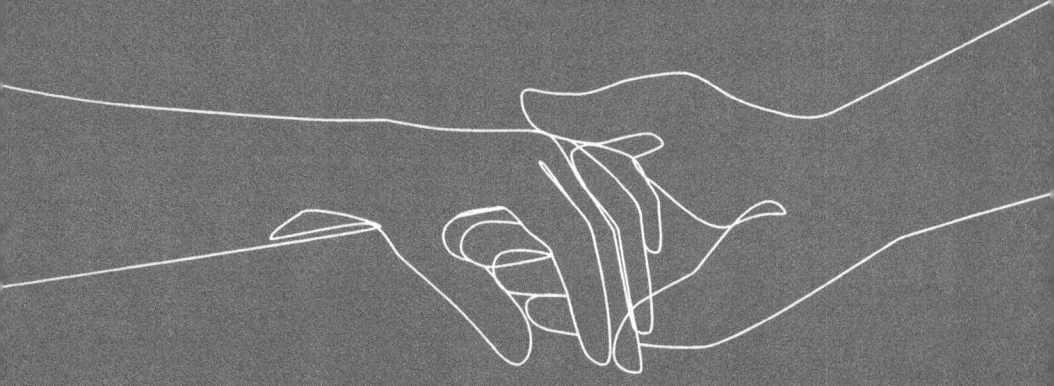

Menopause isn't just the women's 'problem' to solve, it affects the whole family unit and should be treated as such.

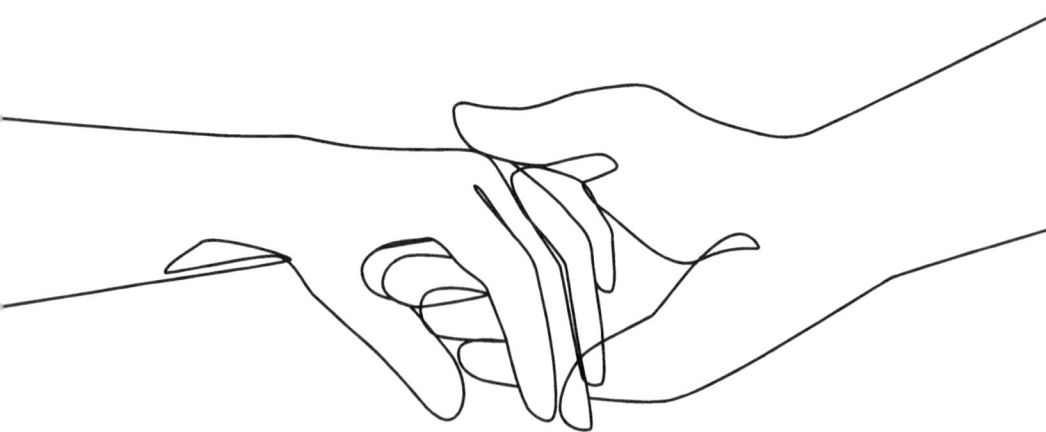

Marriage Through Menopause

When we go through menopause, often the main thing men see is that the woman they love is changing – and that's understandably unsettling. She is more moody, more irritable, sleeping way less, crying more, and doesn't want to be touched let alone intimate. This can leave them feeling helpless, confused and even rejected. They feel as if they are not wanted or needed in a loving way, which isn't the case at all. We definitely don't want our partners to feel like this and we don't do it intentionally. But when our hormones are wreaking havoc on who we used to be, it's hard to see through it.

When a woman reaches menopause, there's often a disconnection between what she is experiencing and what her partner can understand. It makes sense, because most partners only know us from the point they met us as a girlfriend, the wife and a mother. What is often forgotten or not understood is that long before these roles, she was a young girl learning how to become a woman. That transformation from girl to woman, which is often awkward, emotional, painful and confusing, was navigated silently for a lot of us. We had to learn how to deal with our shifting hormones and the emotional and physical changes that come along with that. So as most of our partners weren't there for our first transition, they now get to see us through another transition – which feels unfamiliar for both of us.

Through all the challenges menopause brings, the inevitable question arises, "How long is this going to last?" Unfortunately, the answer is one that none of us like. But it's not a problem for our partners to 'fix', it's a transformation that they need to support us through. When she hears from you, "How long?", what she's really hearing is, "When will you be normal again? When will you stop being so emotional? When will you go back to being you?" But we aren't going back – this is the new version of us that has just been brought to the surface. The one who has been dug deep for a long time and is finally coming out. The one where we get to evolve with power, and if you support her through this evolution, it can be the best thing that happens to her.

> **We don't need to be fixed. We need patience when she is tired, silence when she needs space, comfort when she feels like a stranger in her own body, and curiosity instead of criticism. We want connection.**

So instead of asking, "How long will it last?", ask her "How are you feeling? What can I do?" And if she seems overwhelmed trying to explain what she needs, use your initiative to figure it out to take the pressure off our already fogged up and overwhelmed systems.

Menopause doesn't have an expiry date, but the support we get can make all the difference. She will remember it, and it will eventually deepen your connection.

All we ask is for love.

You can't help with our sleepless nights or our body changing or the hot flashes or the sudden waves of emotion that catch us off guard. We don't need the flowers (although they are appreciated), or the solutions and explanations, we just need real, patient, unwavering love. The type of love that says, "I'm here, I see you and I'm not going anywhere."

Without love, the journey becomes too complicated and heavy, and this is where many relationships suffer under the weight of misunderstanding. In fact, the divorce rate increases around the age of menopause…

This brings me to the one word a lot of partners think when it comes to women: "Crazy." We hear it *all* the time, but it's especially potent around menopause. Our partners have most likely known us for twenty plus years and then all of a sudden, we are identified as "crazy". This makes us question ourselves, and think, *are we? Is this how the kids feel too? No, surely I can't be going crazy?*

My husband Pip was speaking to a friend and asked him how he was going. The friend responded that he had separated from his wife. Pip responded with, "Why? Is she going through menopause?" His friend said, "Yes she has gone crazy on me."

Instead of taking an empathetic approach to a huge hormonal change, it's easier to just say that we are crazy. It comes across as dismissive, insensitive and even offensive, especially when we already know we feel like shit and aren't acting like ourselves. When we express strong emotions, we get told we're "overreacting" or our children tell us that "it's not that deep."

When we are being dismissed this way, it can lead to self-doubt, anxiety or depression, so it's important to have a compassionate, patient and understanding partner who is going to help you through this phase. Like any problem that occurs during marriage, the question arises: "Are we going to work through this together or not?"

Last week, I hadn't slept very well for two nights in a row, so I caved and turned on the TV. I came across a series called *Four Seasons*, which has Tina Fey in it. I love her as an actress and she also produced it, so I was pretty excited to watch it. It follows three middle-aged couples who have been married for decades and go on a holiday altogether each season. Without giving too many spoilers, the show explores how long-term relationships change and evolve over time. It didn't directly mention menopause, but it was obvious that it played a role in how a few of the relationships had changed in the most recent years, especially the relationship breakdown at the forefront of the show. One of the men decides he wants to divorce his wife because she has gotten 'boring' (aka probably depressed and low-energy from menopause) and he wants someone who is younger, more adventurous and full of life. On the other hand, one of the other couples shows the flipside where although they are arguing more and their relationship goes through some rough patches, they ultimately decide that they still love each other and want to be together.

The moral of the story for me was that there are men in the world who aren't prepared to ride the roller coaster of menopause and deal with the major changes that happen with their wives, and then there are the men who buckle in for the journey and stay by their wife's side. For the former category, I get it because at this point in their lives, a lot of men are at their peak of how good they feel within themselves and want their partner to reflect that. There is no right or wrong, but it comes down to which kind of man you want to be in your relationship.

The seasons of each episode in the show symbolise a stage of life or relationship evolution: spring (new beginnings), summer (thriving), autumn (unravelling), and winter (loss or renewal). Menopause is like autumn and winter – a time when things feel unfamiliar and there are identity shifts and emotional energy changes. When a woman begins to change physically and emotionally, her partner either grows with her or he begins to seek emotional withdrawal. Some lean in with empathy and others pull back, mocking or minimising the changes and labelling us crazy.

The series shows us how no relationship stays the same and pretending it will only leads to resentment or distance. Menopause is not the end but a transition that requires presence, effort and most of all love. It can go two ways: it can be a wake-up call or a missed opportunity for deeper connection.

It is likely the biggest test of your relationship, and while it's super challenging, it's definitely not impossible. If love, effort and respect lead the way, life will be good. We don't want to just be 'tolerated', we want to be chosen again and again, but we won't beg for it. Not now, not ever. It's a matter of through thick or thin, till death do us part. I always ask the question to my husband, "God forbid if I were sick with some sort of illness, how would that be any different?" With menopause, the pain we carry is within ourselves and can't be seen physically as such, but that doesn't make it any less life altering.

Menopause: A Husband's Awakening

When I met my wife Wendy, she was the miracle that walked into my life. I could see that she was extremely intelligent, talented and caring, and she brought warmth into my life. At a time when I was still trying to find my place in the world, she saw something in me that I didn't yet see in myself. Her belief gave me drive. Her calm gave me direction.

Wendy showed me what love was really about – family values, togetherness and the importance of celebrating life. Christmas, birthdays, milestones – things I overlooked – became moments to cherish. She taught me the true meaning of connection and how powerful family love can be when it's nurtured and appreciated.

My dream was always simple: to marry, have kids, and give my wife and family a lifestyle where we could have and do whatever we wanted, whenever we wanted – no expenses spared. I was dead set on providing a quality life for them. That was my mission, my purpose, my fuel.

We married on the 7th of October, 2001. Twenty-four years later and we have a beautiful family with three girls and one boy. They are our world, our chaos, our pride.

Fast forward to 2025... and If I can be completely honest, our house feels different. My three daughters are all synced with their monthly cycles, and when you throw in menopause, this is something I was not ready for.

Menopause didn't just take my wife away for the time being – it replaced her with someone who was fighting her own invisible battle, and I had no idea how to reach her. When I did try with physical affection, it wasn't reciprocated. This was my idea of intimacy and connection, and it took me a long time to learn that she was yearning for a different type.

Some mornings it feels like I'm walking through an emotional minefield. One wrong comment, one sarcastic remark, and boom, the energy in the house shifts. Other days, it's laughter, music and dancing in the kitchen like old times. It's unpredictable, and I've learned that no amount of logic or reasoning works when hormones are in charge.

No one talks about how menopause affects men. How it leaves you confused, rejected and wondering where your partner went. You start to question yourself, your worth and whether the love you built your life around still exists. My mind would wander to the worst places – questioning my role as a husband. There was a massive fear of losing Wendy. I couldn't help feeling that we weren't the same couple we once were.

After about 2 years of feeling this way and numerous conversations with Wendy, I finally began to understand how menopause was affecting both her and our family. I knew very little about menopause, but I soon learned it can turn a world upside down. It did exactly that to ours. It affected every corner of our family life. The mood swings, the distance, the silence – they all started to affect our daily rhythm. The kids couldn't understand it, and honestly, neither could I. I held onto the hope that once menopause was 'finished', we would return to normal. I kept my eyes firmly grounded on this imaginary finish line; however, I soon realised that's exactly what it was: imaginary. Menopause isn't a phase; it's a transition.

As time went on and the 'bury-my-head-in-the-sand' approach clearly wasn't working, we opted to see a marriage counsellor. We even tried one-on-one sessions separately and I tried to work on myself so that I could show up better for her. I went to the gym more and started investing in my mental health. Even so, it wasn't helping – we were on a road to destruction and there were no answers in sight.

I never imagined my wife of 24 years would be experiencing something so foreign to me as a husband and a man. It scared me, but at the same time, I knew I had to grow with her and I realised I needed to educate myself more about menopause – to understand what was really happening, not just to Wendy, but to all of us. I started listening to podcasts, reading articles and researching facts. I wanted to know what this stage of life actually meant for her – emotionally, mentally and physically.

I also joined a men's group. It was an online forum where men from all over Australia come together to openly share their stories and lessons about relationships, fatherhood and menopause. That's when it hit me: no one is immune to it. Every man in that group had their own version of the same struggle — unable to truly understand and support their partners in the way they needed to be.

It didn't fix everything overnight, but for the first time, I realised I wasn't crazy — I was just uneducated about something that affects every family in one way or another.

I started seeing a psychologist more regularly — she was a highly educated woman who helped me with my personal healing and sorting out the pain of my past. She dug deep. She didn't just listen; she felt it. We both cried during some of those sessions. They were heavy, raw and at times confronting, but she became my saviour at a time when I was most vulnerable. For the first time, I was unpacking years of suppressed trauma, fear and emotional buildup I didn't even know I was carrying. This allowed me to reflect more powerfully on how I had been showing up in my relationship with Wendy and how my behaviours were intensifying the changes Wendy was already going through. By reflecting on myself, I was able to identify ways I could change to adapt to this new reality and create a more peaceful home.

From March 2023 to now, our relationship has improved but it's not perfect. We are steady. We talk a lot more. I try to provide more obvious gratitude for everything she does and be more proactive, rather than just assume she will do it. I've learned to let things go, give her space when she needs it, and provide intimacy and connection in the ways she needs it: deep conversation, quality time and understanding. There's a point when you realise the love you once knew isn't the same anymore. It's not gone; it's just changed shape. The hugs are shorter. The intimacy is different. The laughter's quieter. The spark you built your life around feels dim.

I used to think love was about fixing things. If something's broken, you roll up your sleeves and make it right. But menopause doesn't work like that. You can't fix hormones, you can't reason with exhaustion, and you can't force connection. Letting go of control has been one of the hardest lessons of my life. What love looks like now is different. I think it's less about passion or excitement anymore and more about patience, commitment and showing up even when it feels hard.

**Love is staying loyal.
Staying calm. Staying patient.**

It's not easy watching the woman you love go through something you can't help her with. You want to reach out, but sometimes that only pushes her further away. So you learn to step back. You learn to listen more than talk. You learn to be still. But you don't always get it right. It's a constant process of learning how to be the person she needs at that time. I help her as much as I can, as I'm fully committed to both Wendy and the kids.

Being a Mother Through Menopause

One afternoon I was having a conversation with my youngest teen, and she looked at me with those wide, honest eyes and said, "Mum, I'm proud of what you're doing… but sometimes we don't get to have you like we used to."

And she was right. She hit me in the heart with her truth. But she wasn't accusing me of anything, she was simply observing what we both knew. Because for so long, my salon was simply a space to do hair and my number one job was always being their mum. But as they grew older and started to be more independent and as I came through menopause, something shifted. It wasn't that I forgot about my kids – far from it. But I did start to pour more of myself into my salon, my brand, and now this book. And in a way, it's been therapeutic. A lifeline. Something that's held me through the storm and given me something just for me. And yet, it comes with its challenges – the guilt, the juggle and the inner conflict of doing something for yourself when you've spent years being everything for everyone else.

I'm forever grateful they're all out there, living their lives, being independent and finding their way, but I do miss them deeply.

Armani just got her license and that one hit me. She is the last of my four to start driving, and it signalled the end of an era. No more school drop-offs. And even though yes, I did feel like a taxi, I do miss those car rides. That's where I got told everything without even asking. Where we would laugh, talk about the drama at school, sing to blaring music. And then, just like that, it's gone. It's another reminder of that empty feeling that sneaks in sometimes – that realisation that I'm not needed in the same way anymore. That's where my brand, my book, and Pip come in, they fill that missing link. Keeping busy and creating: that's where I feel most alive.

But you know what's been the most beautiful part? Seeing my kids batting for me. Cheering me on. Believing in me. They're behind me, 100%. And that support has meant more to me than I could ever explain.

My Children's Perspective

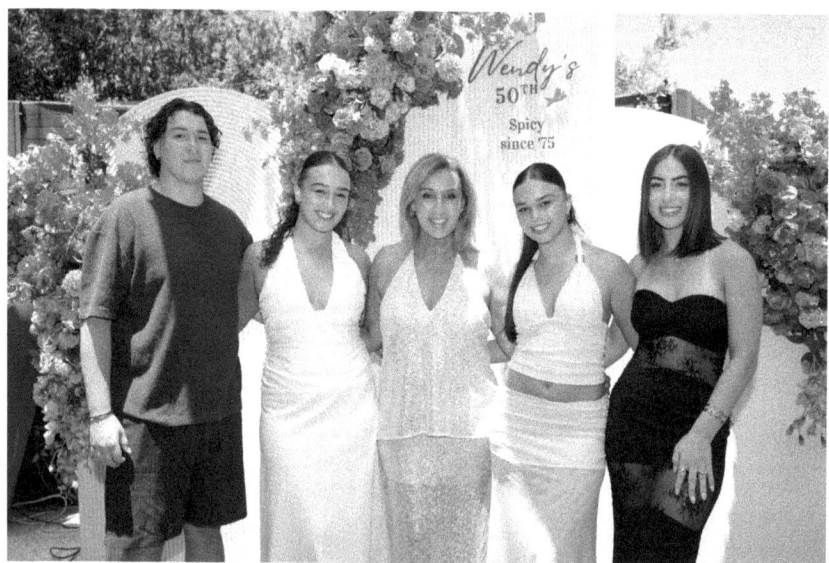

Nataya

Growing up, my mum was always our rock... the calm in the chaos, the one who seemed to have everything under control. But when menopause began, things slowly started to change, and as her children, we felt it too.

At first, we didn't really understand what was happening. One moment she'd be laughing with us, and the next she'd snap over something small or retreat to her room in tears. We learned to tread carefully, walking on eggshells at times, not because she was angry or mean, but because we could sense she was struggling with something deeper, something she couldn't always explain.

There were days when her energy was low, when she seemed distant or exhausted, and we missed the version of her who was always so full of life. But then there were also moments of incredible closeness, times when she opened up and let us see her vulnerability. Those moments taught us empathy, patience, and what real strength looks like.

Menopause didn't just affect her; it affected our whole family dynamic. It tested our understanding, our communication and our ability to support each other. But it also brought us closer. We learned that love doesn't always look like perfection — sometimes it's messy, emotional and raw.

Looking back now, I realise how brave she was. She was navigating physical changes, emotional swings and a loss of control over her own body, all while still showing up for us. Watching her go through menopause reminded us that even the strongest people need care and compassion too.

It wasn't always easy, but it taught us resilience, empathy and the power of unconditional love — lessons that will stay with us for life.

Levi

Being the backbone of our household and the glue that holds us all together, Mum has always been the one keeping us steady — the strength in the storm and the heartbeat of our home.

When the first signs of change came, it caught us off guard. We'd never seen this side of her before. One moment she'd be laughing with us, and the next she'd be exhausted, overwhelmed and on the edge of tears. Days blurred together — some were low for her while ours stayed high — and it took time for us to truly understand what she was going through.

There were moments she opened up, tears falling as she whispered that she felt she wasn't good enough. She was tired. She couldn't sleep. She was drained. But even in those moments of weakness, I saw a different kind of strength in her.

As a family, we had to learn what menopause really means. We had to listen and actually make an effort to understand. Especially me and Dad, two people who will never know what it feels like but can only do our best to stand beside her with patience and love.

Through it all, we've seen the real Wendy Naumovski — the woman who never gives up, even when her tank is empty and the fuel light's been on for miles. The woman who walks through dark tunnels and somehow still finds the light. The woman who gives every last piece of herself to the people she loves.

Mum has a heart bigger than anyone I know and a drive that refuses to fade. Watching her still show up, still give and still love while fighting one of the toughest emotional and physical battles is something I'll never forget.

We see you, Mum. We love you. And we're so proud of the woman you are — in every version, in every season.

Caprice

Being 18 and watching my mum go through menopause has been one of the most unexpected lessons of my life. Growing up, I saw her as this unshakeable force: strong, steady, always in control. But menopause has shown me a different, more human side of her, right as I'm figuring out who I am too. Some days, it honestly feels like I'm living inside a climate disaster movie. One minute she's freezing cold, and the next she's opening every window like we're inside a boiler room. Sometimes she'll start a sentence and forget what she was saying halfway through, and we just sit there in silence waiting for her delayed response because it's all you can do.

There's a funny, chaotic rhythm to it that you eventually learn to move with. But underneath all the humour is something much deeper. Menopause doesn't just change her body, it affects her emotions, her energy, her sleep and the way she sees herself. There are days when she's exhausted before the morning even begins, days when she feels overwhelmed for reasons she can't quite explain, and quiet moments where I can tell she's trying to understand what's happening within her own body. Those moments have changed the way I see her.

I don't just see my mum anymore: I see a woman going through something powerful and difficult, someone who still shows up, still tries, still loves even when she doesn't feel her best. And that kind of strength is so different from the invincible image I had of her growing up. It's softer, more vulnerable, and somehow even braver. This whole experience has taught me patience, compassion and how to support someone without always having the answers. I've learned not to take things personally, to give space when she needs it, and to be present when she doesn't want to be alone. She's adjusting to a new stage of life, and I'm adjusting to adulthood. Strangely, our two transitions meet in the middle, teaching us both how to communicate and understand each other in new ways. If anything, menopause has brought us closer. I see her more clearly now, not just as my mum, but as a woman navigating a major shift with courage, humour and honesty. I hope she knows I notice her strength in the small moments, the hard days and the ones where she laughs through the chaos.

Menopause might be her journey, but in a way, it's become ours. And I'm right beside her – learning, supporting and growing with her through every change.

Armani

Watching my mum go through menopause has been both challenging and eye-opening for me as a 17-year-old. I knew that something in her had shifted, but I just wasn't really sure what. She wasn't the same person she used to be. There have been tough times where her moods changed suddenly, and I didn't always understand what she was feeling. Sometimes she would get upset or emotional over things that never used to bother her, and it was hard not to take it personally. There were times when we clashed and there were moments that really tested me. Like when she'd snap over something small or go completely silent when I needed her. I used to get frustrated and think she didn't care, but deep down I knew she was just trying to hold herself together.

I started realising that menopause isn't just about getting older, it's about your body changing in ways you can't control, your emotions shifting without reason, and trying to find yourself again through it all. I could see the exhaustion in her eyes, the moments where she wanted to be strong but didn't have the energy to pretend anymore, or when I felt helpless because I couldn't fix what she was feeling. Even through all the mood swings, hot flashes, and sleepless nights, she still showed up for me, took me to school, made my lunch every morning and kept being the mum who loves and protects me even though she was exhausted 24/7. I've also seen her soften in some ways. Over time, she became more reserved and quiet, often putting her headphones in and shutting everyone out. She'd say that we wouldn't understand, and in those moments, it felt like she was drifting away from us. I knew she didn't mean to push us away, but it felt like she was building a wall around herself to cope with everything happening inside her body and mind, lost in her own thoughts.

It was painful to watch because I wanted to help, but I didn't know how to? This was the hardest part. I'd get frustrated or emotional too, because it felt like I was losing the version of my mum I grew up with – the loud, funny, talkative one who always filled the house with energy and asked everyday after school how my day was. But at the same time, I started to realise that she was still there, just dealing with something massive that I couldn't fully see because I was still so young and didn't understand.

The more I learned about menopause, the more I understood how much it takes out of a person physically, mentally and emotionally. I've learned to be more patient and gentle with her, to listen instead of react, and to give her space when she needs it. With my mum experiencing menopause, it has also made me more independent in ways I never expected. I used to rely on my mum for everything: making my lunch, washing my clothes and ironing my school uniform for the next day. But when I saw how much she was going through, I knew I needed to start taking care of myself more. At first, it was hard. I'd forget to make my lunch or realise I didn't have a clean shirt for school or a creased top and she would yell at me about it but I would reply ,"Well you didn't do it so I had to" – not knowing how much she was going through at the time and how much pressure I was putting on her when I was capable of doing those things myself.

Menopause has tested our relationship in so many ways. When we would get into fights, I would always bring up, "This stupid menopause is doing my head-in" and she would get so sensitive about it and we then wouldn't talk for days. I felt like sometimes I just didn't have that mum figure from her anymore. I'd come home wanting to talk or needing advice, and she'd be too tired or quiet to respond or be asleep on the couch at 4pm. For me, it's been a huge lesson in patience and understanding. I've seen my mum's strength in a whole new way, not the kind that shouts all the time, but the kind that survives quietly. My understanding of menopause has definitely grown, and I've learned that it's so much more than just a 'phase' women go through. It's an emotional, physical and mental journey that completely changes a person, and I've seen that firsthand through my mum. Watching her struggle, shut down and slowly rebuild herself has opened my eyes to how strong she truly is. It has made me more patient and more appreciative of how much she does for me and our family. I've grown in ways I never expected, becoming more independent and more understanding of my mum. I no longer just see her as my mum, but as a woman who has faced and is still facing one of the hardest chapters of her life.

Seeing her face menopause every day has made me realise just how strong she is inside and out. No matter how difficult things got, she never stopped trying and I'll always be so proud of her. I will never forget what this time has taught me and what it really means to be there for a loved one through their hardest moments. I love and cherish my mum so much and I'm so proud of how she has handled her time facing menopause.

PART 5

Moving into the Future
with Wisdom and Wholeness

If you feel like you're falling apart, know that you're actually becoming whole.

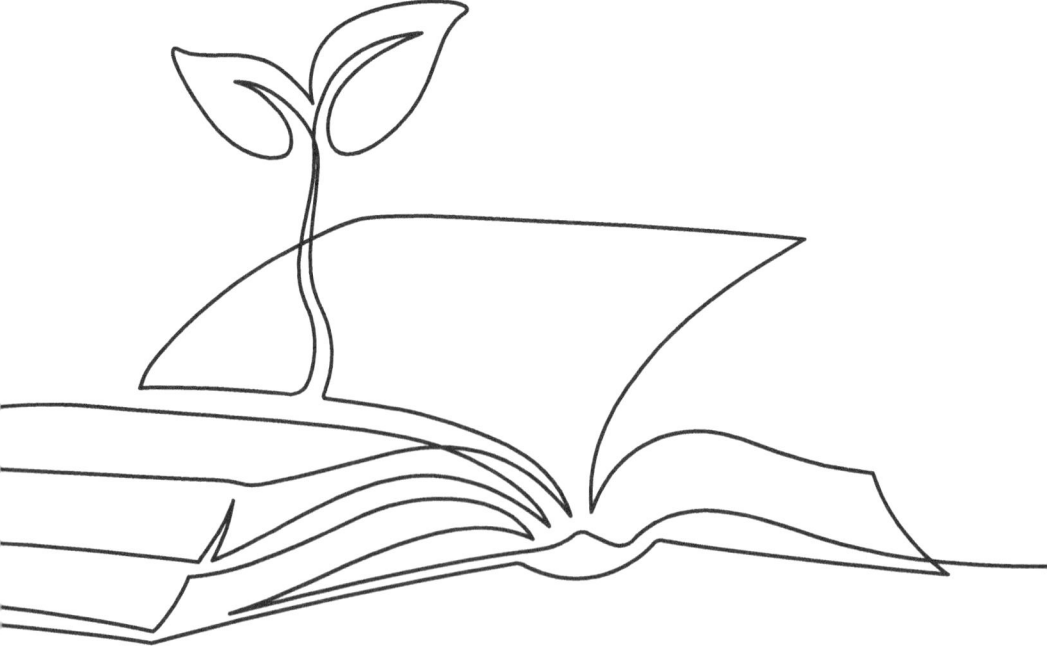

Healing My Inner Child

I often think back to when I was around 10 or 11 years old. I can't remember the exact age, but I remember the feeling in my body as though it was yesterday. My mum would leave early in the morning for work, often before the sun came up. Her day started at 5am, and that meant mine did too. My aunty would drop my little cousins at our house, and with my sister being 9 years younger than me, the responsibility fell on me to make breakfast for my sister and cousins and ensure everyone was dressed and ready before I had to leave for school myself around 8 or 8:15.

This was not once a week or an occasional duty – it was a few days a week. It became normal for me to carry adult responsibility while still a child. I look at my own children now and imagine them having to do what I did at that age, and it feels almost unthinkable. But at the time, it didn't feel like a choice. I simply got up and did it. There were no questions asked, no arguing, no chance to say "I'm too tired" or "this isn't fair." All I knew was that my mum needed to get to work, and I needed to help make that happen.

What strikes me now, as I look back through the lens of menopause, is how much I learned to adapt and how much I was conditioned to suppress my own needs. If I was tired, that was too bad. If I wanted to spend time with friends or sleep in, it wasn't an option.

> My role was always to hold
> things together, to make sure
> others were okay.

As my sister grew older, those responsibilities grew too. I would walk her to and from school, look after her during school holidays, clean the house, cook dinner, and in between all of that, I held a casual job to earn my own money. Childhood for me was never about freedom or exploration. It was about responsibility, sacrifice and stepping into a role that wasn't meant for me yet.

Fridays were always special though. Tate, my dad, worked away in the bush welding pipes, and there was no way my mum was able to contact him. So during the week, it was just Mum, my brother, sister and me. But on Fridays, we would wait eagerly for Tate to come home – listening out at 4pm for the sound of his car coming into the driveway. After he got home, he would sometimes take us to a toy shop not far from our house called Wonderland. To a child, it really was a wonderland – shelves that seemed to stretch forever, aisles lined with toys that made our eyes light up as we walked in and that whispered promises of joy and possibility.

My dad would say, "You've got this much money – buy what you like." It was his way of rewarding us for helping Mum, for keeping things together while he was away. Those moments felt like treasure, not just because of what we got to bring home, but because it was time spent with him, a gesture that made us feel seen and appreciated.

One particular Friday, I chose a doll. She wore a pink dress, had long blonde hair and big brown eyes. She was so pretty and I had to have her. I spent hours brushing her hair, changing her outfits, and carefully placing her in the middle of my bed. Every morning when I made my bed, I set her in the same spot, perfectly positioned. When I came home from school, I would know instantly if anyone had been in my room because she would be in a slightly different position. Mum was good at covering up for my sister, who would always deny touching her, but I always knew if she was moved.

Alongside that doll, my room itself was my sanctuary. I had a Queen Anne bedroom set: white and elegant, with a dresser, cupboard and bedhead that made me feel like a princess. Messiness and disorder unsettled me, so I would clean my room, rearrange it and decorate it until I felt it was perfect. I wrote in there, I drew in there, and I spent hours writing in my diary. We are encouraged to write in journals today, but it was a natural thing for me back then to write in my diary, as well as draw. I spent hours drawing cartoon characters or I would go to the park and draw the trees and landscape. When I bought a stereo with my very first paycheck, my room fully became my own little world. I'd listen to the top 40 on the radio and wait to press record to tape the latest songs.

As I moved into my pre-teen years, things started shifting. My doll stayed on my bed, but I started craving something different:

stories, answers, realness. That's when books entered my life. Books didn't just take my attention… they completely took over.

And of course, it all started with Judy Blume. She was real. She said things how they were. No sugar-coating, no pretending. Her books felt like someone finally opened a window and let the truth in. It was like she understood what girls my age were going through before we even knew how to explain it.

Then came *Sweet Valley High*… and honestly, that's when reading became a full obsession. *Sweet Valley High* wasn't just a book series. It was *the* thing. If you didn't read it, you weren't cool. It was all the hype. Everyone was either Team Jessica or Team Elizabeth. We lived for their drama – the boys, the friendships, the popular girls, the chaos of high school life. And those boys… always sporty, always the dream!

Finishing a book and going to school the next day was the best part. We'd meet up and talk about it, but not give away too much in case someone was behind. And you *never* skipped to the next number. That was basically a crime! We waited for each one like our life depended on it.

Every Friday night, my dad and I would go to Kmart – our weekly ritual had changed from the toystore to the book store. I can still picture it perfectly: walking through those sliding doors, heading straight to the book section near the stationery, and seeing a crowd of girls waiting to grab the newest *Sweet Valley High* book. It was like a sport – push, shove, reach, grab. And if you were slow? Too bad, someone else got it. You had to be quick to grab the book you were up to reading or it would go, but Fridays were when the shelf would get restocked and the new books added.

The excitement was insane. That feeling of getting the next volume… Honestly, it felt like Christmas morning. I couldn't wait to get home, jump into bed, and start reading. At first, Dad only let me buy one book. He probably thought it would last me a week. But when he saw how fast I got through them, it became our thing. Every Friday he'd ask, "What number are you up to now?" And then he started surprising me – coming home with two, sometimes three, because he knew I'd fly through them.

I remember hitting book 54. Don't ask me how many they made – I still don't know – but that number stuck. It felt like an achievement. Those books shaped us more than we realised. They taught us about friendships, jealousy, crushes, heartbreak, loyalty – all the things we were experiencing but didn't know how to explain yet.

And here I am now, decades later, experiencing menopause and realising how deeply those early years shaped who I am. As a child, I learned quickly not to complain, not to resist, not to ask for help. I learned that my value was tied to how well I could hold everything together. I learned that everything costs money, that belongings are to be cherished, and that gratitude must come before comparison. Friends had more, some had less, but I was taught to appreciate what I had. I feel like we are living in such a materialistic time that we forget to stop and think about what we have and what we appreciate. My parents would only upgrade something if it was broken and unrepairable, whereas today, we change not because it's broken, but just because we want to.

There was a time my brother and I decided we wanted bigger bikes – you know that feeling when you're a kid and you have outgrown your bike. One Australia Day, our family went to the Skyshow. There were thousands of people there, the smell of barbecues was in the air, and there were fireworks lighting up the sky. When it was over, everyone started packing up their blankets and chairs, ready to head home. Just as we were getting ready to leave, my dad handed each of us a garbage bag. He said, "Here you go. You said you wanted new bikes."

We looked at him, completely confused and honestly, a bit embarrassed. But he meant it. So off we went, the two of us walking through the crowds, picking up aluminum cans that people had left behind. We walked with our heads down, embarrassed to be seen. Everyone else was heading home, and there we were, collecting cans. But as the bags started filling up, I started to get it. My dad wasn't trying to make us feel small; he was teaching us something big.

He wanted us to understand that if you want something, you have to put in the work. Nothing just shows up. You create it. You earn it. And sometimes, the path to what you want doesn't always look glamorous.

And now, going through menopause, I think about it even more.

This stage of life has a way of grounding you. It strips away ego, perfection and what you thought life was supposed to look like. It reminds you that the best things – strength, peace, confidence – are things you build yourself. Sometimes, from pieces you've had to pick up again.

Menopause can feel uncomfortable and confronting. But underneath it all, it's about rediscovering your value. Seeing what's still beautiful, still useful, still strong.

Dad wasn't just handing us garbage bags that night. He was showing us how to take action when we want something to change. And that's what this stage of life asks of us – to do the work, to show up and to believe we're still capable of building dreams.

> It's not about approval now,
> it's about being seen.

I particularly cherished my doll because it represented recognition. It was my dad's way of saying, "I see you. I appreciate what you've done." As a little girl, I always looked for validation from my dad, and this continued on up until I was in my early 20s. His words – a compliment, a recognition of the work I'd done, or a "Thanks for dinner, it was delicious" – meant everything. They were proof that I was someone worth noticing.

Now, as a grown woman, a wife, and a mother, I don't need that validation anymore. But I'll admit that it still matters. It's not about approval; it's about being seen. As women, especially in menopause, we often feel the opposite: invisible, overlooked, no longer rewarded or even acknowledged for the unseen labour we carry.

> I still have that deep desire to
> feel valued, not just for what
> I do, but for who I am.

The longing I felt as a child for that recognition resurfaces now, as I still have that deep desire to feel valued, not just for what I do, but for who I am. It's been buried for so long as I always put others before me, but menopause demands we slow down and come face to face with who we truly are. Then our family thinks we are crazy because of our outbursts in rage, but no one looks deeper to see what's behind it. It feels like a confrontation with all the parts of ourselves that were silenced, and for me, that was the part that was allowed to think about themselves and to ask for help.

Unpacking the Years of Suppressed Emotions

The anger and frustration I feel during menopause – the sudden irritability, the pissed off thoughts that seem 'small' – aren't just hormonal, it's layered with decades of unspoken truth. It's the ten-year-old in me who never got to say this isn't fair. It's the teenager who spent her holidays babysitting instead of being carefree. It's the young woman who thought sacrifice was normal.

One time my parents decided they would go up north for a holiday and take my sister with them, so my brother and I decided to rebel in the best way we knew how – to get the phone book out and call our friends to tell them we were having a party. We had no driver's licenses and obviously weren't old enough to buy alcohol, but we had a taxi to take us to the shop to get chips and dips and uncles that we conned into buying us alcohol.

The party went well. It was the first time I saw my brother drunk, and we had our friends stay over. And as I was brought up to be tidy, the next morning I blew a whistle, got everyone up, and we cleaned the backyard. We removed every bit of rubbish – every can and every cigarette butt – so there were no traces of a party. *What party?*

We did not want to be home when my parents got back because we were so scared of getting into trouble, so we went to our uncle's house. Did our parents find out? Yep, they sure did. One place we forgot to check was the letterbox and there was a can in there. On top of that, my cleaning of course wasn't up to Mum's standards, so she was re-mopping the floor when we got home.

During menopause, we yearn to push boundaries, just like teenagers. But instead of that rebellion coming in the form of a house party, we have the desire to stop pretending, to let go of perfection, and to finally live without guilt. The rebellion isn't against our parents this time, but against the roles, rules and expectations that no longer serve us. Menopause uncovers those buried feelings and brings them into the light. It has a way of stripping away the masks we've worn, and suddenly, the emotions I suppressed as a child – the exhaustion, the unfairness, the longing for freedom – rise up.

At first, they came out as anger. Anger at my family, at myself, even at the world. But as I sat with them, I saw that beneath the anger was grief. Grief for the childhood I never really had. Grief for the girl who carried so much without being asked if she could. And yet, alongside that grief is gratitude. Gratitude for the resilience I built, for the independence I gained, for the lessons that made me who I am today. What I see now is how deeply generational these patterns are. My mum didn't know any better. She had been raised the same way – expected to care for her siblings, run the household, and sacrifice childhood freedoms for responsibility. She had no teen life either – she went from household chores to meeting my dad and then she started her life very naive as she hadn't experienced anything. She passed that expectation onto me without questioning it, just as her parents had done to her.

Go Easy on Your Mum

To say that growing up in a European home was strict would be a huge understatement. Love often came wrapped in control. Protection sounded like criticism. Care looked like fear. They loved us deeply, but they also carried generations of worry about reputation, safety and what people might say.

If I so much as mentioned going out with friends, going for a drive, or out to a club, it was like I'd said something criminal. Mum would look at me like a disappointment and I couldn't work out what I had done wrong. It was all so foreign to her. Every time I walked out the door, I felt guilty, like I was doing something wrong just for wanting to live a little. And every time I came home, whether I was on time or late, she was angry. As a result, Mum and I clashed a lot in my teens. I felt like she was constantly watching me – my own private detective. I couldn't breathe without her questioning where I was or who I was with. At the time, I thought she didn't trust me. But looking back, I can see now that it wasn't about trust. It was fear.

Dad was different. The first time I came home drunk, instead of yelling, he just handed me a blanket and a bucket. That was it. No lecture. No drama. Just quiet understanding. Dad would say, "Go easy on your mum. This is all new to her. She never got to do what you're doing."

And he was right. Mum never had the freedom I did. She never went out with friends, never had sleepovers, drives, or nights that turned into stories. Her world was small, structured, and built around responsibility. So when she saw me stepping into my free, independent life, it triggered something she didn't understand. I used to resent her for being so strict, but now I understand she was only doing what she knew. She wasn't trying to stop me from living, she was trying to keep me safe in a world she didn't understand.

Now, as a woman moving through menopause, I see my mum so differently. She's the 'cool' grandma to my kids, the relaxed one that I wish I had as a mum. But I'm grateful that my kids get this version of her. Back then, I thought she was just overbearing. Now I see a woman who never had the chance to be a girl. Someone who went from daughter to wife to mother without ever having the space to discover who she was.

Menopause does something similar. It forces you to look at yourself again, but this time not through anyone else's lens. It's confronting, but also freeing. You start asking, *who am I now? What do I want?*

And I can't help but think that maybe if Mum had been given that space, she would've found her own freedom too.

So when I think back to those years and to all our clashes, I hear Dad's words again: "Go easy on your mum." And I do. Because I see her now not just as my mother, but as a woman – one who carried fear, duty and love all at once.

Menopause has taught me that our mothers didn't have the language, the tools or the freedom to express what they felt. But we do. And maybe that's how the cycle changes – not through blame, but through understanding.

Breaking the Cycle

I look back now on that little girl who woke up before dawn to feed and dress children that weren't hers, who never argued, who just kept going, and I want to tell her that it's okay to rest. It's okay to want more. It's okay to be a child.

> And now that I'm in this stage of life, it's forced me to stop, reflect, and decide what patterns we will continue and what we will end.

Growing up, I was used to hearing "no" before I even asked, and I learned to stop trying. When I was younger, I wanted to be a journalist because I loved writing and art, and I loved dancing and wanted to pursue it more seriously. I still remember the day the letter arrived holding my dreams. I had auditioned for a particular dance program at a nearby school, and my heart was pounding with hope when I tore open the envelope. The first word that greeted me was, "Congratulations." I had done it. This was my ultimate dream and I was so excited. I went and shared my good news with my parents, expecting the same excitement to spill back to me. But instead, the answer was a big fat "no."

My dream was shut down, not because I wasn't a good enough dancer, but because I had to take my sister to and from school and that was more important. I sat in my room and cried and thought life was so unfair. I was devastated. By year 12 when the dance team at my school was preparing for a tour to New Zealand, I braced myself for the same disappointment. But this time, my parents had no option but to let me go, as the guilt got the better of them. My parents' fear had silenced that dream with a firm "no". For years, I carried the weight of what could have been.

But entering menopause has lit a fire in me: I will not pass this down to my children. Instead, I choose to show them courage, resilience and the importance of dreams. I get to watch my three girls dance on stage, and let's just say, I am one proud mumma. They do it not because I force them to, but because they choose it and they love to dance.

Menopause holds space for all the 'yeses' I have always wanted. Whether it's the freedom I never had or rediscovering my passions to be able to put myself first without an apology. I carry both truths, the ache of all my deferred dreams and the knowledge that there are endless possibilities because it's never too late.

> **Menopause became my wake-up call – a reminder that it's never too late to break cycles.**

Breaking cycles for me means looking at my daughters and choosing differently. It means allowing them to be children for as long as they can, encouraging them to rest, to play, to explore. It means not asking them to sacrifice their freedom in the same way I did. I learned this as I watched my eldest daughter grow up, as I realised that I had passed some fear down onto her. I have apologised to her, as I can now see I was doing the same as my mum. During menopause, I have learned to accept things that affected her and looked at my decision-making process differently. I changed my way of parenting real quick so I didn't make that mistake with her. I am grateful that I was mindful to see it before it was too late.

By choosing differently for them, I am healing something in myself too. And that means learning to put myself first without guilt. It means acknowledging that rest is not weakness, that asking for help is not failure, and that my worth is not tied to how much I sacrifice for others. It means giving myself permission to feel – anger, grief, joy, gratitude – all of it. And most of all, owning it if I was in the wrong, without a debate. Writing this book has allowed me to process everything, let it go and move forward.

Forgiveness plays a powerful role here. Forgiveness not only for my mum, who was only doing what she knew, but also for myself – for the years I carried resentment. Menopause has taught me that holding onto the past weighs heavier than any hot flush or sleepless night. If I hadn't learned to heal and forgive, I would still be clinging to the anger of all the things I was never allowed to pursue. The emotional turbulence of menopause forced me to confront those wounds, and forgiveness became my medicine. Forgiveness doesn't mean forgetting. It means acknowledging the pain, understanding its origins, and choosing not to let it define me. I can be grateful for the strength my upbringing gave me while also grieving what it cost me. I can carry both. And in menopause, this balance becomes essential. Grief grounds me, while gratitude releases me.

Silent Suffering Is So Last Era

I was thinking about my mum and my grandmother the other day. We say they were strong, that they just "got on with it" when it came to menopause. They were strong, no doubt about it, but I couldn't help but wonder, did they "get on with it" or did they just suffer in silence? Did they even know what they were going through?

People say life was simpler back then, less stressful. And in some ways, maybe it was. I remember my own childhood – one after-school activity for an hour that we would walk to, dinner on the table at 6pm sharp, and then all of us showered and watched *Home and Away* together before bedtime.

Compare that to my life with four young kids, which consisted of being a taxi service from 4pm to 7:30pm, juggling different sports bags, snacks, and sometimes even dinner in the car. It's a world away from how I grew up. Women are expected to work, raise a family, and do it all with a smile. But where we differ from our mum's generation is that it's no longer taboo to speak about "women's things".

Let's be real, our generation grew up in a world where you didn't even mention the word 'period' in front of your dad, let alone see commercials relating to it. It was a hushed conversation or hidden, something never spoken about openly. So, it's no surprise that menopause was completely off the table. It was *the* big, unspoken secret.

My mother went through menopause without a word. Like it didn't exist. She was brought up to "just get on with it", and this is how she grew into a strong, resilient woman with a lack of communication. The advice she gave to me as a child was "don't worry about it", and this is the advice she still gives me to this day. And because she never spoke about it, I never knew what to expect and was nonchalant about what was coming.

Did they really "get on with it" or did they just suffer in silence?

In school, we were taught about our periods and the female reproductive system. Later, we had sex education, which focused on contraception, pregnancy prevention and safe sex. By high school, the information went deeper, with discussions around the pill, alcohol and drugs.

When we become mothers, we have access to antenatal classes – sessions preparing us for delivery, books, videos and endless information about pregnancy itself. There was even some mention of postpartum, what our hormones go through after birth. But menopause? Silence. Nothing. Not in health class. Not in antenatal classes. Not even a pamphlet slipped into the pile when you first start bleeding, or when you fall pregnant, or after you give birth. Nothing to prepare us for what comes at the other end of fertility. It's the bookend to our reproductive lives, the final chapter, and we're expected to just stumble into it blindfolded. That has major consequences for our relationship with both ourselves and others.

When our daughters come to us and say, "Mum, I just got my period," we respond with awareness and care. We check in: "Are you okay? Do you need anything?" As a family, we know to tread gently during that time – to give space for moods, to expect a few changes for a few days, as having three girls in sync each month can make for a hectic household. It becomes something we can tolerate, because we understand it. We've been prepared for it.

But menopause is different. When peri arrives, there's no announcement, no warning, no marker like a first period. It blows in like a gust of wind you weren't expecting, and suddenly everything changes. The moods, the hot flushes, the exhaustion, the brain fog. And unlike a period, it doesn't last a few days and the people around us don't know what to expect or how to handle this new version of you. That's the hardest part: the silence and the surprise. Families don't have the prep. Husbands, children, and even we as mothers are caught off guard. We don't know how long it will last, when it will ease, or how to navigate it together. It can throw a household into turmoil, and you look around and think *wtf is happening to me?*

We've been prepared for everything *except* menopause.

If there had been education, if menopause had been treated with the same seriousness as periods, pregnancy and postpartum, we could have moved forward prepared, armed with knowledge instead of confusion. We could prepare our families with the same kind of awareness and it would take away the shame, the secrecy and the frustration, replacing it with understanding and connection. We as mothers and wives don't want to be fixed, we want you to be by our side. My favourite saying is, "It's not about you. I'm trying to find out about myself."

The knowledge we build through our own experiences shouldn't stop with us. It should ripple forward, breaking the cycle of silence, ensuring the next generation isn't left in the dark. It was too late for our mums and too late for us – let's make sure it's not too late for our daughters, as well as our sons to help their wives deal with it all a bit better.

Outside of educating women, two of the most important places to foster understanding and knowledge are in the home with partners and in the workplace.

Educating Men About Menopause

Women are raised to be resilient, to endure, to suffer in silence, and just get on with it. Whereas men are raised to be providers, protectors, and to dismiss what they don't understand. It's a dynamic that has played out for generations, across many cultures, and it's one that comes to a head during menopause.

So, what happens when a woman starts her journey into perimenopause? When she's confused, exhausted, and overwhelmed, and the man she loves has no idea how to react? Too often, he says the wrong thing. "It's not that bad," he might say, trying to fix a problem he doesn't understand. And just like that, the woman who has given everything to her family feels completely and utterly alone. Even with a family as big as mine, one thing I felt the most was alone, and it scared me.

I started to notice more and more how lonely I felt, but it turns out I wasn't the only one feeling that. I was out with friends, and one of my dearest friends confided in me that she was struggling with perimenopause. She felt disconnected from her feminine side, from her emotions, from her husband. Later that night, I saw her husband make a crude joke at her expense. He didn't mean to be offensive, but I saw the pain in her eyes. She was embarrassed, and quite frankly, devastated. He played the macho guy while she sank with humiliation. I suppose this wouldn't be a bother if you were 21, but at this different stage of our lives, it sounds like an ick.

My husband saw it too. I discreetly went up to him and said, "Don't you think you should say something?" He agreed, so he pulled his friend aside and had a quiet word. He didn't shame or judge him. He just explained how those words can land when a woman is feeling vulnerable. He told him that this isn't a phase to be joked about; it's a life transition that requires support, not ridicule. I was impressed with Pip and how he addressed it.

And you know what? It worked. The next time we saw them, something had shifted. The husband was gentler, more attentive. He listened more. He showed up with more care. It was a small change, but we could see he made her feel more comfortable and she could be more genuine.

> And it all came down to
> one thing: education.

Her husband wasn't a bad guy; he just wasn't educated. No one had ever taught him about menopause, and he wasn't the only one. The only thing most men were ever taught about women's bodies was how to not get pregnant.

That's why we have to talk about it. We have to break the cycle of silence and ignorance. We have to teach our sons, our husbands, our brothers, and our friends what it means to be a woman in this world. We have to teach them about periods, about pregnancy, about postpartum, and yes, about menopause.

Because menopause isn't just a woman's journey, it's a family affair. We are there for our husband's major life changes, but often one of the biggest things that happens to a woman is overlooked. However, when men understand menopause, women suffer less. When men stand by our side, not as bystanders, but as active participants, our relationships evolve. When we educate our sons, our daughters will walk through this phase with more grace, security and understanding than we ever had.

Menopause in the Workplace

We need to stop the silent epidemic that happens across all workplaces: in offices, classrooms, salons, hospitals and boardrooms. In Australia, 29.7% of working women will retire under the age of 55 each year, matching the average age of onset for perimenopause and menopause. While there are a myriad of reasons for this early retirement, there are conservative estimates that at least 10% is due to menopause – the total lost income and superannuation earnings for this portion lands at $17 billion. Anecdotally, 83% of respondents to a research survey said their work was negatively affected by menopause, and almost 50% said they considered retiring early or taking a leave of absence due to menopause symptoms.[2]

Despite this, menopause is not spoken about or even considered in the workplace, and when it is, the question that is often quick to rise is, "What do you mean? It's only menopause – I'm sure you'll be okay." But are we? It doesn't come with sick leave or reasonable adjustments. But should it? It's the same consideration for extra sick leave for periods. I used to get very sick when I had periods, with cramps so intense it would cause vomiting and fainting. Yet I was too embarrassed to call in sick because it wasn't a 'real' reason to be off with sick leave. On one occasion, I was really ill but I didn't want to let my clients down, so I did the 12-hour shift and would sit in the staffroom in between clients feeling faint and weak. It was so heavy that I bled through my dress and had to put a second apron on the back to continue working. I was raised to believe that work came before everything else. No matter how sick I felt, I was taught to get up, get dressed and show up. Illness, especially period pain, wasn't a valid reason to stay at home, it was a challenge to overcome. I was reminded often that I should be grateful I even had a job, and the best way to prove that gratitude was through loyalty and endurance. Rest was a luxury, not a right. My upbringing shaped me into someone resilient, determined and dependable, but it also taught me to ignore my body until it would start screaming. The message was clear: strength meant pushing the fark through and not complaining.

Every day, millions of women work through period pain and millions work through menopause.

Hot flashes behind the desk, brain fog in meetings, mood swings, and low quality sleep disrupting energy levels. And through it all, we keep going, smiling, pushing through and most of all showing up. Because this is what we have been taught. But the big question is: *at what cost?*

Menopause doesn't wait until we are ready to make space in our lives for this change. It comes crashing in when women are peaking in their careers, raising teenagers, or supporting aging and sick parents. We make room for pregnancy, for parenting and even mental health days, but menopause is almost invisible.

As if we haven't been through enough, we get tested once again and we learn to keep juggling both mentally and physically. "It's nothing – you will get through it, everyone goes through it." Well yes, everyone does go through it, and this is why it deserves space not silence. We don't see the women navigating their usual responsibilities with the added complication of physical symptoms that are changing who they are.

A perfect example is that when I was in year 7, I had a teacher who I really liked in year 6 and was excited to be in her class again. However, within the space of a year, she went from being the nicest teacher to this moody angry woman who I ended up disliking. We clashed often, and the more I disliked her, the more I challenged her and the more she punished me. She constantly picked on me, and it got so bad, my mum went and had a meeting with her to discuss why we were clashing. She admitted to Mum that she was going through "a change of life", as they used to call it, and she was not managing it well. I was confused at the time, what the hell is a *change of life*? I didn't get it and I never once thought it was related to menopause. I feel bad now – obviously I didn't know what she was going through at the time and Mum didn't really explain to me what it actually meant. I still had no idea what it was all about, but Mum just said to go easy on her, tone it down and not challenge her. Maybe I'm now getting a little payback for what I did to her!

As for someone like me who has a physically demanding job, it is the hardest on my body. I stand for hours, have no time to eat or take a break, get dizzy often, and deal with swollen and painful legs. I'm lucky enough to be in a position where I run my own business, so I've adjusted my hours to suit my new needs. However, not many women have this flexibility and freedom to work around their symptoms, and it impacts their ability to perform at work. We don't need to be treated as fragile or 'broken', but we want to be understood and most of all heard. We want to feel empowered to work and supported to keep working in a way that is beneficial to both us and the companies we work for.

I believe the first step to workplace understanding is to provide awareness training, where all staff (but especially managers and HR) get a better understanding of the challenges women are facing during perimenopause and menopause. A lot of places do workplace health and safety, diversity and mental health training, so adding a menopause module into the latter category could do wonders for understanding. It would also benefit women in general if their husbands/partners had this training at work and could apply that knowledge to them as well.

> **We don't need to be treated as fragile or 'broken', but we want to be understood and most of all heard.**

We've been conditioned to believe that if we just work harder, lean in more, or act more like our male counterparts, we'll succeed. But that's a lie. We're trying to fit ourselves into a mould that was never meant for us, and it's breaking us. We're afraid to speak up, afraid of being judged, afraid of being seen as less capable, less committed, or worse, "too emotional". So, we suffer in silence, just like our mothers and grandmothers did, perpetuating a cycle of invisibility.

> **When you're told to "power through" or "just deal with it," it reinforces the idea that your natural biological processes are a weakness, something to be hidden or ashamed of.**

This isn't just about physical discomfort, though believe me, that's a huge part of it. It's about the subtle ways the system undermines us. When you're struggling with sleep and you're expected to be sharp and articulate in an early morning meeting, it's not just inconvenient; it's a setup for failure. When brain fog makes you second-guess every decision and the culture demands unwavering confidence, it chips away at your self-worth.

It's essential to think about ways that other types of people can thrive – which would be beneficial to everyone involved. It would keep more women in the workplace and with more capability and stronger work ethics. It's about honouring decades of experiences, leadership, emotional intelligence and care that menopausal women bring instead of just dismissing them because they can't fit themselves into the standard mould of work anymore.

Full Circle Moments

During a family trip to Melbourne, we stayed in a small town called Kyneton, and not far from there was Mount Macedon. One day we drove to see the cross at its highest point, and then to Hanging Rock – made famous by the haunting story *Picnic at Hanging Rock,* a book I'd read in my early teens. I remember the eerie beauty of the place, not knowing that decades later, it would hold a different kind of meaning for me.

Fast forward to when I'm 49 years old and I'm back in Mount Macedon, but this time not as a wide-eyed teenager – now as a woman writing her own story. I was there for a publishing retreat at Dean Manor with my husband by my side. As I sat in that beautiful setting, working on the pages of my book, it hit me: this is what they mean when they say life is one big circle.

Back in March 2022, I had a tarot reading with my friend Kristy, who has a gift for seeing beyond what's obvious. At that time, I was just starting to navigate my own journey through menopause. I wasn't looking too deeply into it yet – just feeling my way through, unsure of what lay ahead.

She spoke of seeing me bringing something out into the world. She saw me educating, standing on a stage and sharing knowledge. I remember thinking, "Yeah, right… what on earth would I have to bring out?" The ideas felt interesting, but I couldn't connect them to my life in any meaningful way. I tucked those words away and moved on.

Two years later, in 2024, I found myself replaying that same recording. But this time, I listened with a completely different lens. As I heard her voice, my heart skipped a beat. Everything she described was now unfolding in my life – my brand, my book, my mission to educate women and hairdressers about menopause and hair health.

I could see it.
I could feel it.
I could be it.

It wasn't magic that made it happen. I don't live my life by waiting for the universe to deliver. But I do believe in visualising what I want, holding that vision, and taking action towards it. That combination – belief and effort – is where the real transformation happens.

That tarot reading didn't give me the answers. It planted a seed. And maybe it took 2 years for me to grow into the person who could see it clearly, but now I know my path: to empower women like me, to give them tools and confidence, and to guide the next generation of hairdressers in understanding and supporting clients through one of the most powerful transitions of their lives.

And this is how I connect my life's journey to menopause – it's all about transitions. Returning to Mount Macedon was both familiar and new, just like each stage of menopause. You step into it thinking you know what to expect – after all, you've been through hormonal changes before: puberty, pregnancy, postnatal shifts. But then, just like walking a path you once knew, you realise things look different now.

Menopause isn't one single moment; it's a series of transformations. Some are subtle. Some hit you like a storm. You shed parts of yourself, revisit old versions of who you were, and discover aspects you didn't know existed.

Just as I stood in the same town decades apart, seeing it through new eyes, menopause has brought me back to parts of myself I thought I'd left behind. Only now, I'm not the girl looking for approval or permission. I'm the woman rewriting my own script, deciding what stays, what goes, and what transforms. And maybe that's the gift in all of this. The full-circle moments remind you that while life may bring you back to familiar places, you arrive there with new wisdom, new strength and a deeper understanding of who you've become.

Signs, Feathers and Ink

I've been reflecting a lot lately, especially as my brand and book start taking shape. Whenever I see a connection or a hint that I'm on the right path, I can't help but ask myself: *Is this a sign?*

Or am I simply looking back and seeing the way my past connects perfectly to where I am now? Maybe it's both. Maybe it's the extra guidance I've been getting from my baba from above – pushing me to keep going, breaking the generational cycle and doing what needs to be done.

The night before my son's 21st, I was setting up and found a feather inside a plastic card box. Just sitting there. Random, yet not random at all. All day long, I had been seeing angel numbers appear: 111, 222, 444. Over and over. Each time, I'd glance upward and say, "Thank you" because I know my baba is with me every step of the way.

Everything I'm doing for my brand and book is for the next generation, but it's also for my mum and for my baba – women who were never truly seen or heard. Baba's favourite saying to me was always: "Ako da bidish zivi i strav." *Do not worry as long as you're healthy and strong.* That's what mattered to her.

Just last week, Pip, the girls, and I (Levi couldn't make it) went to light a candle for his dad at the cemetery as it's been 10 years since he passed. Afterwards, I said I'd go and light a candle for my dedo (grandad). Pip looked at me and said, "What about your baba?" And my heart dropped – I'd forgotten.

Walking to their graves and seeing them side by side hit me hard. I had a lump in my throat standing there, as I realised this was the first time I'd been there with them both gone. It still doesn't feel real. Part of me still thinks Baba's at the nursing home. I didn't go as often as I should've because I found it hard not having Baba's house to go to anymore, the place that always felt like home. Her garden full of greens, the smell of cooking drifting through the air, jars of chilli lined up in the shed, and her sitting on the verandah waiting for me to come through the side gate. Those memories are stitched into me.

That morning, after visiting them, my irritation lifted. It grounded me. It was my moment of peace, like visiting my own sanctuary. While the thought of going to the cemetery is eerie, once I am there, I feel a sense of calmness.

And now I've decided that her words will be my next tattoo – a permanent reminder of her wisdom and the strength she saw in me.

I'd wanted tattoos since I was a teenager, but was I allowed? Absolutely not. My dad told me that if I got one, I'd never be able to give blood. And I believed him. All those years, I thought tattoos meant something wrong or dangerous – at least in his eyes. But when I went through perimenopause, the rebel in me came out. I thought, *Why not now?* So I got my first tattoo when my daughter also got hers for her 21st birthday. Sitting in the chair, I asked the artist about my dad's 'no blood donation' rule and she just laughed – definitely not true. Turns out, my dad just wanted his daughters to have 'clean skin'.

When we went to Nataya's birthday lunch, I felt like a little girl again, hiding my tattoo from my dad. Nataya ended up showing him before I did, because grandparents always respond differently to grandchildren. To my shock, when I finally showed mine and explained the meaning behind it, my dad said, "I really like it – it looks good." I almost fell off my chair.

His approval meant more to me than I wanted to admit. Should I have cared that much? Maybe not. But it made me feel lighter. Seen. Validated.

Now, I think – why did I wait so long? I could have done it years before I did. But maybe the timing had to be right, a few years before my 50th, to claim something for myself. To make it meaningful. To make it mine.

My Dad – Keeper of Memories

A few years ago, my Dad told me he still had the whole set of *Sweet Valley High* books. He'd kept them all this time. I honestly didn't believe him until he recently showed up with the box full of them looking brand new.

When I opened that box, I felt like I was right back in Kmart. All the excitement, all the Friday nights, all the moments that were just me and him – it all came rushing back. I showed my girls thinking maybe they'd feel some spark, but of course they didn't. And why would they? Their world is completely different. They have unlimited options; we only had *Sweet Valley High* and we treasured it. In the mix of all the books were my diaries that he also kept for me. I would spend hours before each school year decorating my diary with cut out words and pictures stuck to it. I cherished them and was so happy to have them back.

But what hit me most wasn't the books… it was the fact that Dad kept them. He looked after them like they were pieces of my childhood he didn't want me to lose.

I thought I was the one collecting books.

But really, he was collecting memories of me.

Now those books sit in my home all lined up perfectly, just like when I first bought them. They're more than stories, they're pieces of my life. Pieces of who I was. Pieces of who my Dad helped me become and grow.

And as I navigate menopause, these books remind me of something simple and comforting: there are parts of me that time can't change.

The little girl who loved stories.

The teenager who raced home to read.

The daughter who adored her dad.

And the father who kept every single book safe… just for me.

It's funny how life circles back. How something from decades ago can suddenly mean something completely different when you hit menopause.

When my hormones started shifting and everything in my mind and body felt unfamiliar, I found myself reaching for comfort. Not the kind you buy or book in, but the kind rooted in who you used to be. The parts of yourself that felt steady, uncomplicated and true. And somehow, *Sweet Valley High* became part of that comfort.

During menopause, so much feels like it's slipping: memory, identity, patience, clarity. You start questioning who you are now compared to who you were before kids, before marriage, before responsibilities. Before the world sat so heavily on your shoulders.

And then one day, my dad showed up with that box with the books he'd kept safe for me. I didn't realise it at the time, but opening that box was like opening a doorway back to myself. Back to the girl who raced down Kmart aisles full of excitement. The girl who couldn't wait to read. The girl whose biggest stress was whether book number 27 would still be in stock. The box still had a strawberry scent to it, and I found the little Strawberry Shortcake figurine tucked in the corner. I wasn't interested in the other characters, just Strawberry Shortcake and her scent was so mesmerising and refreshing.

Menopause can strip you down. It can make you feel lost in your own skin. But holding those books reminded me that deep inside all the chaos, the exhaustion, the brain fog and the emotional waves was still a girl who feels things deeply, who finds joy easily, who loves stories and routine and connection.

These books aren't just nostalgic. They're grounding.

When I hold them now, I'm reminded that I've lived through so many versions of myself: daughter, teen, young woman, mother, business owner. And I'm still evolving. Menopause isn't an ending. It's another version of me being born.

And sometimes, to feel steady again, all you need is something familiar in your hands. Something that reminds you of simpler times. Something that brings you back to your roots.

For me, it was *Sweet Valley High*.

A reminder that the girl I was still exists inside the woman I'm becoming. A reminder that old memories can feel like a warm hug. A reminder that joy can return in the simplest ways.

And most of all, a reminder of the beautiful softness of life cycles – how things come back to you when you need them most, wrapped in nostalgia, love and the tender fingerprints of someone who kept them safe just for you.

The New Way

This year, I turn 50. Half a century. That number doesn't roll off the tongue easily. It lands with weight. Not just because of the age, but because of everything it represents. It's not a 'just another candle' moment, it's layered. Emotional. Defiant. Proud. Tender.

As the number 50 approaches, there's a little girl in me that starts tugging at my sleeve. She wants to laugh louder, dance wildly, and not give two fucks about how she looks or if she said something stupid. She wants to be free again. Unfiltered. Joyful. And sometimes I feel her bursting out and I think, *Yes, that's me*. That's always been me. But other times, I quiet her down.

Growing up, I was the girl who always had to make excuses to not attend what I was invited to – not because I didn't want to go, but because I wasn't allowed to. While others were going to parties, sleepovers or spontaneous beach days, I was home watching life from the sidelines. As a result, I learned early to quiet my own desires, to dim that part of me that longed to be seen and free.

Somewhere along the way, that became a pattern that followed me into adulthood.

As the years rolled on, I became everything to everyone else. But I lost touch with the girl who once wanted to laugh until her stomach hurt, dance without guilt, and live without asking for permission. When menopause began to weave its way into my life, it didn't just bring physical changes, it brought a mirror that forced me to look at who I had become – and who I had left behind.

So when my high school group decided that we'd spend a few days in Rottnest to celebrate turning 50, something inside me lit up. It felt like a calling back to the version of me that I had tucked away. The 'old me'. The one who had been waiting quietly for decades.

Rottnest became a moment in time that bridged the gap between my past and present. The island gave us space to laugh again like schoolgirls, to tell stories we hadn't told in years, to play games that reminded us of who we used to be. There was exercise, laughter, food and a lightness that I hadn't felt in so long.

For the first time, I didn't have to ask anyone's permission to go either. I didn't have to justify my joy or explain my absence. I simply went.

And that freedom… It felt like a victory.

Standing there, with the ocean breeze against my skin and the sound of my friends' laughter in the air, I realised how much I had missed being seen just as Wendy. The woman who loves connection, who craves laughter, who feels alive when surrounded by stories and shared memories.

Menopause, in a strange and beautiful way, had given me that gift: the courage to reconnect, to take up space again and to reclaim joy without apology.

That weekend will stay with me forever. It wasn't just a

getaway, it was a celebration of womanhood, friendship and the power of rediscovering ourselves at a time when society often tells us we're fading.

But we're not fading, quite the opposite actually. We're finally being seen, and not for what we give, but for who we are. And maybe, just maybe, that's what growing into ourselves really means.

The world tells us to hide this chapter – I say we rewrite it

I saw a video the other day and it stopped me in my tracks. "Having four kids means nearly 25 years of your life with children – and four of those you were pregnant. So when you see your mum being a little wild and free, let her. She deserves to be her again." That really resonated with me. I've given so much of myself over the years – time, energy, care and sacrifice. And now I want to find the parts of me I packed away while I was busy being everything for everyone else.

And then there's the mirror… Let's be honest. As much as I try to own it, part of me looks in the mirror and thinks, *Whoa*. The body I see has changed. The skin, the shape, the energy – it's all evolving. Yes, I'm probably too harsh on myself and yes, I'd probably be just as happy sliding under the table on my birthday and letting it pass quietly, no fuss, no big deal.

But turning 50 while going through menopause feels like standing at the edge of something unknown – like you're stepping onto the other side of something big. The world tells us 50 is 'older', but I remember my mum at 50. She was already a grandma for the second time. She wore that role with pride. And for a while, I thought that's what 50 was supposed to look like. But now that it's my turn, it feels different. I don't want to be defined by the roles I play – I want to be reminded of how I feel, how I love, how I show up. I just want to be happy again.

> **I built a brand and a business, raised a family, and now I'm embracing the most honest version of me – in menopause.**

In a world where unexpected loss is around every corner, I don't take this lightly. I'm reminded of the saying that aging is a privilege. I'm here. I've made it. Through babies and business, joy and heartbreak, rage and reinvention. Through every sleepless night, every stretch mark, every self-doubt, every triumph. And I get to celebrate it with my husband, who's been by my side through it all, and with my beautiful kids, who have watched me evolve, fall apart, rebuild and rise again.

So let this birthday go off with a bang. Not because I want attention, but because I want to honour this body. This life.

Turning 50 is a badge of honour. It's proof that I'm still here, still growing, still dreaming. Still *becoming*.

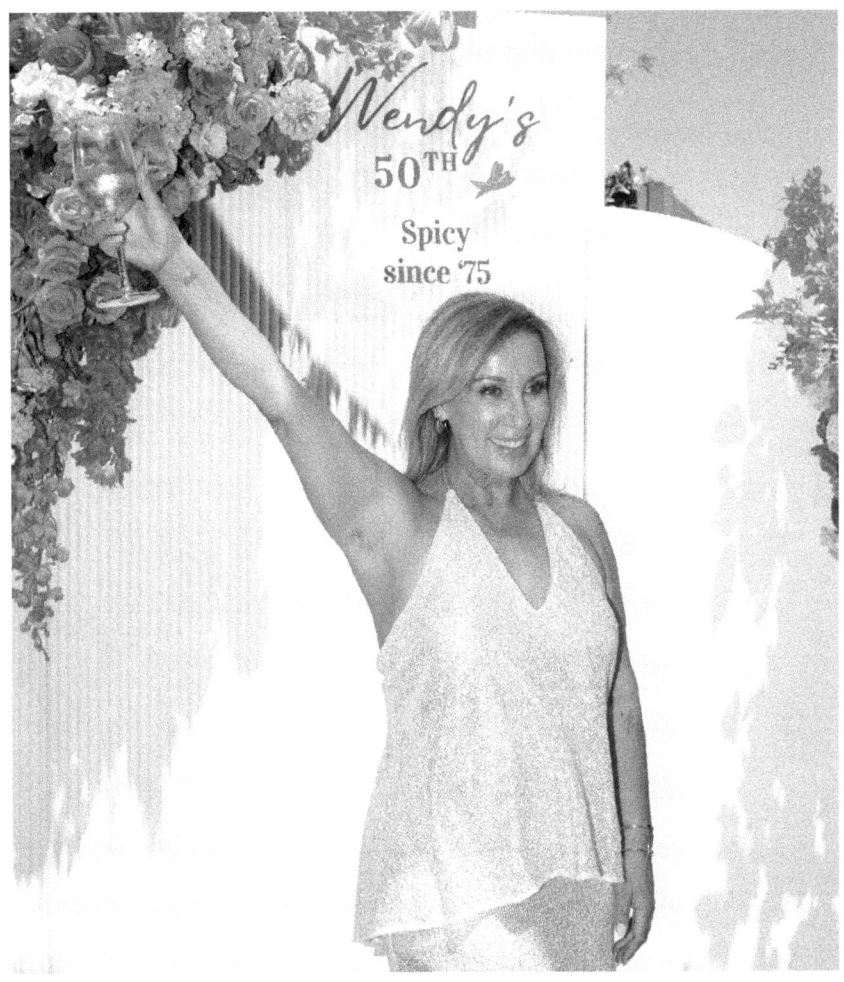

About the Author

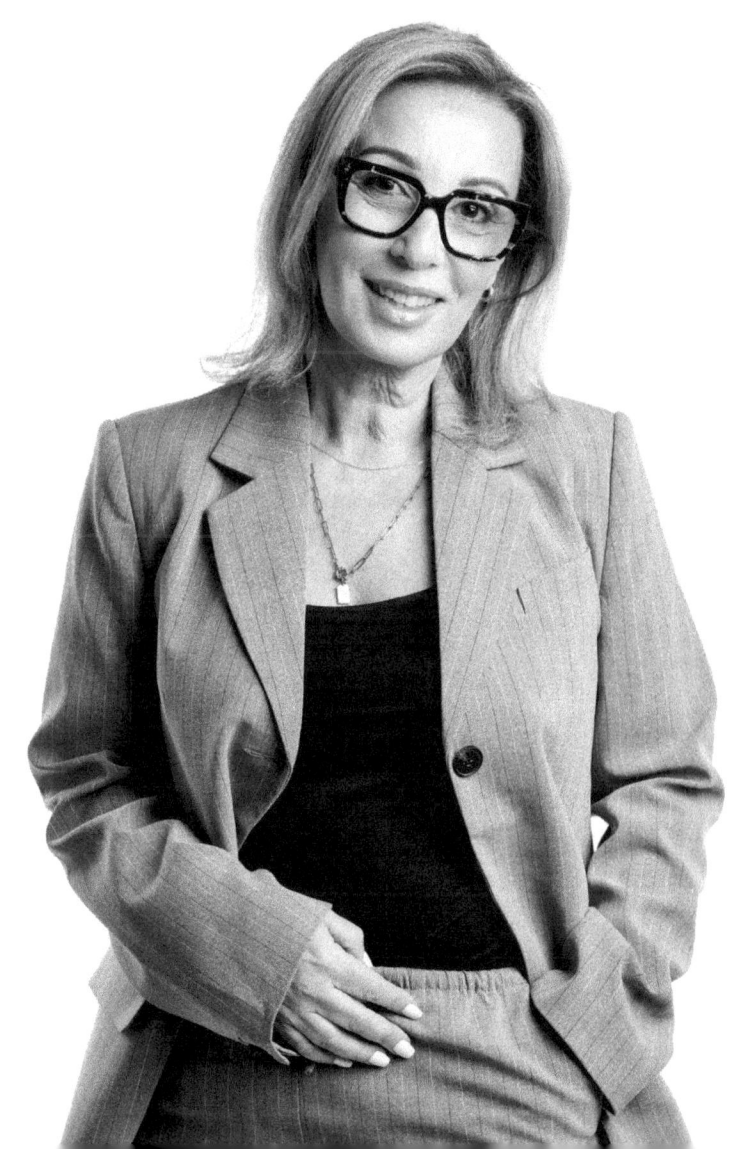

Wendy Naumovski has built her life around helping others feel beautiful – but it wasn't until she went through menopause that she learned what beauty truly means.

With over 30 years of experience as a hair and makeup artist and salon owner, Wendy has seen firsthand how women evolve through every stage of life. Behind the chair, she's heard their stories of love, motherhood, identity and the quiet changes that come with time. When her own body and spirit began to change, she turned inward, exploring the emotional layers of menopause with honesty and grace.

Her book was born from that place – a space between exhaustion and awakening, where she began to understand that menopause isn't a loss, but a return to self. Through her writing, Wendy hopes to give women permission to pause, to care for themselves deeply and to embrace this chapter with tenderness.

She lives in Western Australia with her husband and their four children, finding joy in family, creativity and the small, meaningful moments that remind her of who she truly is. She is entering the next chapter of her life as the founder of Wendy the Brand – a movement and product range created to support women through menopause with understanding, science and soul.

Connect With Me

Wendy the Brand has been created to help women turn their menopause experience from purely surviving to thriving.

Scan the QR code below to find out more, connect with Wendy, and browse the hair products that have been designed especially for menopausal women.

wendythebrand.com

instagram.com/wendy_the_brand

AUDIOBOOK

Great news! *Wendy Talks Menopause* is also available in audio format. Jump onto your favourite audiobook platform now and check it out.

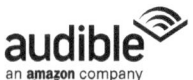 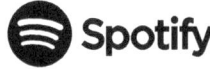

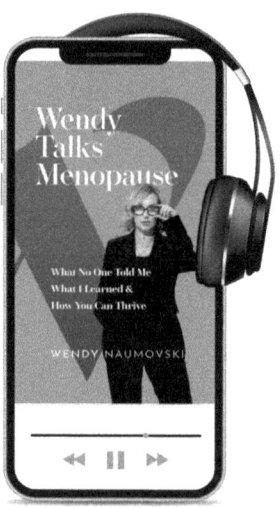

Acknowledgements

To my beloved Baba, whose strength and love continue to guide me every day. It was through her that I learned the true meaning of resilience – to be strong and to heal at the same time. She showed me what grace looks like in pain and how love can live even in silence. It was her spirit that gave me the courage to break the generational chains, to rediscover who I am, and to finally find my voice – to be seen, heard and free. Every page of this book carries a piece of her light.

To my parents, I am forever grateful for how you raised me. You taught me resilience, hard work and the strength to never give up. It's because of you that I am what I have become today. I now see that your fears were your way of keeping me safe, and though your choices sometimes came from pain, I now understand that you did the best you could with what you knew with love. I forgive the past, and I thank you, because it is through your journey that I found mine. I'm grateful that I get to live out what I've always wanted to do, even if it came later in life. I now do it with understanding, compassion and strength – the kind that can only come from healing. I thank you for the love that shaped me, and I carry forward only the strength you gave me.

To my husband, Pip – my anchor through the waves. Thank you for standing beside me with patience, love and understanding. Together we grew and we learnt along the way. You grew to embrace my changes, even when I was learning to embrace them myself and even though it wasn't the easiest. You kept trying and never gave up on me nor us. Thank you for holding space for me as I grew, evolved and became who I was always meant to be. The more I grew, you grew too. Your support gave me the courage to share my truth.

To my beautiful children, thank you for loving me through every chapter of transformation. I know at times it was confusing, watching your mother shift, heal and rediscover herself. But through your love and acceptance, you gave me strength to keep going. You have been my greatest teachers in grace, patience and unconditional love. Just as it wasn't easy for me, it was confusing for you all to be introduced to menopause, but we have always stuck like glue as a family and we became even closer and stronger as a unit over time. The best thing you have all done is never give up on me as your mum.

To Susan and her incredible team at Dean Publishing, thank you for guiding me through this world as a first-time author. From editing to marketing to publishing, your care and dedication made every step feel supported. The Dean Manor retreat was an experience I will never forget for both Pip and me. It gave us a glimpse into the heart and intention that lives behind every page, every call, every moment of creation.

To Daniel Mostyn, thank you for always keeping me focused on my vision, for your honesty, and for reminding me what's possible. Your belief in me helped me see this journey through to the end.

And to the beautiful souls and their small businesses who walked beside me in my healing journey, many are mentioned within these pages. I am forever grateful. Your kindness, understanding, and gentle energy helped me heal with ease and grace. You reminded me that healing is a collective energy – one built on love, connection and community.

This book is more than words, it's a reflection of every moment, every tear, every lesson and every act of love that has shaped me.

May this be a reminder that your voice matters, your story has power, and it's never too late to rise, to be seen, to be heard, and to become who you were always meant to be.

With love and gratitude,
Wendy xx

Endnotes

1. Koçak DY and Varişoğlu Y (2022) "The effect of music therapy on menopausal symptoms and depression: a randomized-controlled study," Menopause the Journal of the North American Menopause Society, 29(5):545–552, doi:10.1097/gme.0000000000001941.

2. Office for Women (2022) 'Impacts of menopause on women's health, workforce participation and economic security,' *Australian Government.*

Reflection Questions

Identity and self

How has menopause changed the way I see myself – not just physically, but emotionally and mentally?

....

....

....

....

....

....

....

....

....

....

....

....

....

....

What parts of me feel lost and what parts feel newly discovered?

Who am I becoming in this next chapter of my life?

Self-compassion and healing

Where have I been the hardest on myself during this transition?

What would it look like to offer myself the same compassion I give others?

What does my body need from me right now – rest, nourishment, patience, boundaries?

Body, hair and self-image

How has my relationship with my body and hair shifted?

What beliefs about beauty, ageing or worth am I ready to let go of?

How can I support my body rather than fight against it?

Emotional and mental wellbeing

What emotions have surprised me most during menopause?

What triggers me and what helps ground me?

How do I currently process stress, and what support do I need more of?

Relationships and boundaries

How has menopause impacted my relationships with my partner, children, friends, or colleagues?

Where do I need clearer boundaries?

Who truly supports me and how can I ask them for what I need?

Motherhood, work and identity

How does experiencing menopause while still raising children affect me?

How has my role in my family or career shifted?

What version of success feels true to me now?

Reclaiming power

What strengths has this season revealed in me?

What am I proud of myself for surviving, navigating or healing?

How can I honour this phase instead of resisting it?

Looking forward

What does my next chapter need to feel like?

What rituals, habits or support strategies do I want to carry forward?

What promise can I make to myself as I move ahead?

www.ingramcontent.com/pod-product-compliance
Lightning Source LLC
LaVergne TN
LVHW051218070526
838200LV00064B/4956